PRAISE

I didn't expect I'd be on the brink of tears after reading a book about ears. There are many deep, powerful messages in this generous book that touch more than the ears and what's between them. This is a book about being human and living your best life. ~Dr. Adele Varcoe

Everyone talks about making sure we stay physically active once we get to over 50, but almost nobody talks about keeping our minds in tip-top condition and how we might go about it. *Your Resilient Brain* bridges the gap, with particular reference to the surprising links between untreated hearing loss and cognitive decline. ~Michael Smith

I love my hearing aids! In 24-hours they have transformed my life and my relationship with my partner Sheryl. Andrew should be awarded an OAM (Medal of the Order of Australia) for services to the hearing impaired and their loved ones. ~Neville Kruss

I had no idea that I'd lost as much as 45% of my hearing in both ears although I certainly knew I had a problem. Being only 60, I didn't want to acknowledge that I had an issue that I thought belonged to the elderly. I was fortunate to attend a talk by Andrew and when I heard about the hearing loss/dementia connection, I immediately made an appointment. The message was further reinforced when I read *Your Resilient Brain*. I was inspired to take more control of my health and implement some of his helpful, scientifically researched lifestyle advice. It's a must read for anyone who cares about their wellbeing into old age. ~Melanie Smith

Published in Australia by
The Hearing and Brain Health Academy
PO Box 785
New Farm QLD 4005
1300 418 852
andrewcampbell@neuaudio.com.au
www.neuaudio.com.au

First published in Australia 2021

National Library of Australia Cataloguing in Publication entry

A catalogue record for this book is available from the National Library of Australia
NATIONAL LIBRARY OF AUSTRALIA

ISBN: 978-0-6452598-0-3 (paperback)
ISBN: 978-0-6452598-1-0 (hardback)

Cover photography by Kine Graffiti
Printed by Ingram Spark

Disclaimer: This book offers health and lifestyle advice and is designed for educational purposes only. You should not rely on this information as a substitute for professional health and medical advice. If you have any health concerns, consult with a health care professional. Don't disregard or delay having medical health care advice from your health care professional because of what you have read in this book.

Your Resilient Brain

How hearing loss impacts cognitive decline, and nine powerful ways to overcome it

Andrew Campbell

Bac Soc Sci (Psych), MClinAud, MACAud

*For the proactive men
and women who wear
their hearing devices
at least 12 hours per day.*

*May this book help
you inspire others
to do the same.*

ABOUT THE AUTHOR

Andrew Campbell is a Masters trained, independent adult rehabilitation specialist audiologist, and a pioneer in the field of cognitive health and hearing. His passion is to help patients return to a fuller participation in life.

As a leader in hearing health care and audiological sciences, Andrew takes a holistic approach to hearing health. He inspires audiences across the world to address their hearing issues to protect the brain and to allow them to live flourishing lives without limitation.

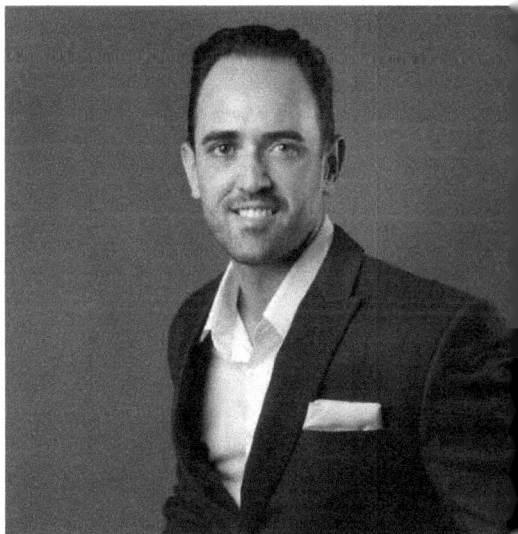

CONTENTS

FOREWORD

As a young professional psychologist, my brain health is of utmost value. I am driven to maintaining a long career, which a decline in hearing and cognitive functioning would no doubt compromise. My knowledge of hearing loss prior to meeting Andrew was limited to the stereotype that it was a condition mainly affecting older people and that treatment requires the use of bulky and unattractive hearing devices.

I discovered that I have congenital hearing loss when after much resistance, I finally had my hearing checked last year by Andrew at his welcoming clinic in Melbourne's Flagstaff Gardens. It was a difficult diagnosis to receive considering I'm a young woman, and the fact that being a psychologist requires optimal hearing to facilitate the best possible outcomes for my clients. I required hearing aids to treat the condition—fortunately the devices are discrete, modern, and barely noticeable.

Since working with Andrew, I have been incredibly surprised to learn that treatment options have significantly improved over the years. Even more exciting has been the functional applications that my hearing aids provide me. They've created substantial improvements in all aspects of my life, particularly with interpersonal communication, which is the foundation upon which my occupation is based.

This understanding was further reinforced when I read Andrew's latest enlightening book, *Your Resilient Brain* where he not only discusses how improving our hearing can also improve our brain health, he identifies several additional methods and strategies that assist in improving our overall mental functioning.

When Andrew discusses the direct implications hearing loss can have on brain health you realize the greater importance of investing in improving your hearing capacity. In particular, the understanding that compromised hearing can influence a person's interpersonal relationships through feelings of isolation and miscommunication, which can significantly reduce mental and cognitive functioning. This is something I found most concerning.

As a psychologist, I am acutely aware of the relationship between various factors including social isolation, increased stress and anxiety, disrupted sleep, poor nutrition and lack of healthy lifestyle choices, and their subsequent impact on our emotional functioning. *Your Resilient Brain* proposes a holistic approach to improving these factors, which may ultimately influence the avoidance of cognitive decline.

Furthermore, it aligns with the growing acceptance and understanding within allied health professions that treatment is most effective when we utilize a multidisciplinary approach that moves from a medical model and towards the recognition that our minds, bodies, behaviors and environment are all interconnected. Therefore, treating one symptom, for example hearing loss with hearing aids, is just one piece of the puzzle. We do greater work when we address all those aspects of a person's existence that are impacted by the symptom, with the realistic aim of achieving optimal management and prevention in the future.

Your Resilient Brain is an insightful and valuable discussion of a variety of factors that we can adopt to improve our overall functioning. Andrew has done an incredible job of collating all of this information into an easy to read, generous, informative publication.

Jill Searle – Clinical Psychologist

Introduction

The brain is mission control for our thoughts and body. It interprets information and controls vital functions such as our heartbeat and breathing. It facilitates thinking and learning. The ears sit either side of the head, but that's not the only connection they have to what goes on in between.

I'm an audiologist so of course I specialize in helping people address their hearing problems. However, what makes my practice unique is that I also consider brain health in relation to hearing issues. The research clearly shows that hearing and cognitive function are very closely associated, and I believe we should work more holistically in that regard. Much of the content of this book does not relate directly to the field of audiology, it is intended to be a diverse account of how we may protect and enhance cognitive function; much of which is interconnected. For a more direct and thorough account of the audiological aspects, you might be interested in my first book *Hearing & Brain Health: Startling links between untreated hearing loss and cognitive decline.*

My goal in founding my company, NeuAudio Hearing and Brain Health, was to help my patients live a life without limitation by helping them remove a substantial barrier to a flourishing life. My mission is to inspire people to understand that hearing is as important as vision. Hearing and vision are broadly considered to be our primary communication senses, however there's a clear tendency to rate our vision as more important. In the Western world, people are around five times more likely to address a vision loss than a hearing loss. When asked whether one would prefer to be deaf or blind, studies consistently show that 83 percent of people would prefer to be blind.

I argue that our hearing is at least equally important because it's a fundamental precursor to our ability to communicate and therefore foster quality relationships. Large scale, longitudinal studies have demonstrated that quality relationships are the most important factor that determine human happiness. By contrast, the least happy people are those who are socially isolated; a situation that is twice as deadly as obesity.

The evidence demonstrating that our brains thrive on connection with other people is overwhelming.

Our capacity to hear well underpins this and yet, most of the time, our vision gets a front row seat. I don't completely understand the rationale behind this cultural blind spot but it most certainly exists, and the ramifications run deep and wide.

In his outstanding book Sapiens: *The Pillars of Civilization*, Professor Yuval Harari, intellectual, historian and philosopher, argues that the core capability that separates human beings from other living creatures is our unique capacity for communication. He states that the Cognitive Revolution occurred between 70,000 to 30,000 years ago, which allowed homo sapiens to communicate with language at a level never before seen. As far as we can tell, only homo sapiens can talk or communicate about things we have never seen, experienced or touched, such as religion, myths, legends, stories and fantasies. These types of communications can lead to collaboration in large numbers in extremely flexible ways.

The COVID-19 crisis forced us to evolve a little more. It took a degree of psychological flexibility, growth and cognitive capacity to cope with a new way of conducting daily life. The new and principal way to keep in touch with family, engage with health care professionals, and to stay engaged with community organizations, was through video conferencing. Even elderly people who had limited experience in using a mobile phone were forced to download an app and navigate a QR code just to get a flat white. If we have limited cognitive ability, these kinds of tasks can be near on impossible, or impossible.

People with hearing loss are at higher risk of suffering from cognitive decline because hearing and memory occupy brain real estate that's intertwined. The stress of hearing loss on memory is now well-researched and has revealed that the degree of hearing loss and cognitive decline is directly proportional; from mild to severe levels the risk increased from 200-500 percent.

In 2017, *The Lancet* medical journal published a study demonstrating that hearing loss is the number one modifiable risk factor for dementia. The terrible irony is that hearing loss is the health issue people are least likely to attend to. However, while treating hearing loss does not guarantee that cognitive decline won't occur (there may be other factors involved), there are plenty of rational and scientifically based reasons that it is one of the best interventions you can take.

The changing world of technology and communications is just one reason to maintain our faculties so we can adapt. How well we deal with change could be a matter of having a growth mindset as opposed to a fixed mindset—terms coined by psychologist Carol S. Dweck. Growth and fixed mindsets describe the underlying beliefs people have about their ability to learn, and their intelligence. A fixed mindset means that you believe intelligence is immovable, so if you're not good at something, it's likely that you believe you'll never be good at it.

"In the fixed mindset, everything is about the outcome. If you fail—or if you're not the best—it's all been wasted. The growth mindset allows people to value what they're doing regardless of the outcome. They're tackling problems, charting new courses, working on important issues. Maybe they haven't found the cure for cancer, but the search was deeply meaningful," writes Carol S. Dweck, in her book, *Mindset: The New Psychology of Success*.

The communication capabilities we inherited from our ancestors, contributes to the richness and nuance that make relationships precious. When people start to lose their hearing, the subtleties associated with intimacy, engagement and humor are stifled and there's a tendency to stick to the basics. Can you pass the butter? Would you like some more potatoes? A life where we are cut-off in some way diminishes what it is to be human.

I'm passionate in my mission to get people to attend to their hearing. The reason I became an audiologist was because I could see the potential to dramatically and measurably change people's lives from their very first appointment. In my regular free seminars on hearing and brain health, I recommend an approach that addresses supplementation, brain training and life-enhancing activities to deal not only with the ears, but what goes on between the ears.

What nearly 20 years of working in the field has shown me is that if you wear your devices full-time and have them adjusted appropriately when needed, there's every reason to suggest you'll hear well for the rest of your life.

As with any other major chronic disorder, be it diabetes, cancer or coronary heart disease, there's immense value in catching and treating these conditions early. It's the same for hearing loss. Much of what's now considered health care could better be described as sick care. Little attention is paid to real prevention, let alone thriving. The medical profession tends to talk about prevention as screening. Too often we wait for a crisis or tragedy before embracing true change. In the case of hearing loss, the true crisis or tragedy occurs when treatment has been delayed to the point where distortion sets in, and clarity becomes a thing of the past. I'm all about treating hearing loss when there's a possibility of restoring what's been lost and preserving residual functionality over the long term so you can retain the faculties to live a full life.

Flourishing – a worthwhile practice

Positive Psychology grew out of the humanistic movement and focuses on achieving a good life. It addresses the ways in which we may flourish, regardless of our circumstances. The focus is on living according to what holds the greatest value to live a meaningful, happy and engaged existence.

Psychologist Martin Seligman established the concept of 'flourishing' within Positive Psychology as the basis of creating a better life. The idea was that instead of focusing on mental illness and negative thinking, the attention would be on what makes life most worth living from an individual and societal level.

Flourishing has several dimensions and one can blossom when one experiences a balanced level of each component. It's not just about happiness and wellbeing, it offers a broader perspective on what it means to feel well and happy. Dr. Seligman developed the PERMA model of five factors that contribute to a flourishing life:

• Positive emotions

• Engagement

• Relationships

• Meaning

• Accomplishments

Flourishing happens when we engage with the outside world and work or activities, enhance our positive emotions, develop meaningful relationships, find meaning and purpose in everything we do and who we are, and apply our gifts and strengths to achieving goals.

According to Positive Psychology theory, you can have a diagnosed mental illness and still flourish. Conversely, a person who hasn't been diagnosed with mental illness can be moribund. That indicates that anyone can find the joy in life no matter their circumstances.

"Flourishing is the product of the pursuit and engagement of an authentic life that brings inner joy and happiness through meeting goals, being connected with life passions, and relishing in accomplishments through the peaks and valleys of life," said Positive psychologist and professor, Dr. Lynn Soots.

Achieving a state of flourishing has many positive impacts including less days off work, clearer life goals, increased resilience, lower risk of cardiovascular disease and decreased chronic illness in ageing.

If you want to flourish, make sure you have a great social support system, and make new friends while strengthening existing relationships. Plan and consciously seek out experiences that are meaningful, fulfilling and fun. Set goals and celebrate your achievements, no matter how small. Never miss an opportunity to laugh—by yourself or with others. Connect with your sense of purpose and meaning and make sure that whatever you do, it is fulfilling and authentic.

Neuroplasticity

It was first discovered in the mid-1900s that the brain was not hardwired and utterly implacable; it constantly changes and has the ability to form new connections when we learn new things. This is called neuroplasticity, which is a dynamic set of processes that can happen at any age. What is fantastic is that we have the power to influence brain changes in a positive way. Even more exciting is that we don't yet know the upper limits.

As an adult rehabilitation specialist audiologist and public educator, I'm in a unique position to gain insights into the greatest concerns of my patients when it comes to their hearing. As it turns out, most are generally more concerned about cognitive decline than they are about the nuisance of hearing loss. Patients frequently ask what else they can do to improve or protect their hearing and brain health. I wrote this book because that question is difficult to address in one sitting.

The resilient brain

A body of psychological literature focuses on the important topic of resilience in dealing with trauma and stress. The ability to be resilient in relation to the ageing process is about staying well, or being disease free regardless of getting old.

Ageing is a complex and multifactorial process that researchers are actively trying to understand. For instance, the question of why some people have brain lesions that are related to Alzheimer's disease, but don't display symptoms.

A fascinating longitudinal study conducted by the University of Minnesota began in 1986. It's known as the Nun Study, which was designed specifically to examine Alzheimer's disease, the most common form of dementia. Researchers followed 678 Catholic sisters of the Sisters of Notre Dame congregation aged between 75–107. Annual cognitive and physical function evaluations were carried out, and with the nuns' permission, they did post mortem neuropathologic evaluations of their brains.

Post-mortem results were surprising. In the case of Sister Matthia who lived to be 105, her brain showed a moderate spread of Alzheimer's; however, she never demonstrated any signs of dementia. Sister Bernadette died of a heart attack at age 85 and her brain autopsy revealed an abundance of the tendrils and growths associated with Alzheimer's. She also showed no sign of mental deterioration or cognitive decline and she sailed through every annual cognitive evaluation.

Clearly, these women had resilient brains and it's generally thought that brain reserve and neuroplasticity were responsible. Brain reserve refers to the capacity of one's brain to overcome the damage done by developing dementia. The nuns' brain reserves somehow gave them the ability to use other resources to compensate for the onset of these diseases.

Recent research supports the concept that the brain can be changed through education and occupation. In other words, our intellectual capability can be protective in relation to dementia or neurodegenerative disease.

Stressful life events can also have a considerable impact on brain function and structure, which can result in the development of some psychiatric disorders. However, not everyone develops those disorders, which indicates that those people are in some way resilient.

Being resilient doesn't mean that you don't experience hard times. It's actually the opposite way around; people who have experienced adversity, emotional pain and trauma are usually the ones who are considered to be resilient. People become resilient because of the challenges; their brains build resilience in response.

In considering resilience, it's not just about the ability to cope, and the spirit and strength to endure the challenges, it's also about our capacity to adapt, bounce back, and grow. This can also be contingent on having a strong sense of self, life-purpose, and optimism for the future.

The resilient brain has increased activation in the left prefrontal cortex (PFC), which is the region involved in things such as executive functioning, memory, regulating our emotions, our personality expression, decision making, and social behavior. It orchestrates our thoughts and actions.

PFC activation can happen 30 times more in a resilient person than someone who is not resilient. This activation can help calm the activity of the amygdala—the place where you experience the flight or fight response. Research shows that the more activity in the left PFC reduces, the more able a person is to turn off negative emotion. Through certain practices such as kindness, compassion to self and others, gratitude, mindfulness mediation and learning, you can build the kind of psychological and physical resilience that will help you flourish no matter what.

Considering your entire being

I recommend taking a more holistic approach, which means attending to all the factors that affect your brain and hearing. This includes mindset, nutrition, and physical and mental/intellectual exercise in addition to addressing any hearing loss. My suggestions are scientifically-based, however it's very important to check with a health practitioner to ensure that any products are completely safe and appropriate for you. Because something is 'natural' doesn't mean it will agree with your state of health or be compatible with any medications you might be taking so please consult appropriate professionals if you're unsure.

I must also point out that, separate perhaps to my small, independent audiology practice, I have absolutely no commercial interest in any of the suggestions outlined here. Plus, there's no clear commercial beneficiary behind most of them. In fact, they are all low or no cost.

My research on cognitive decline and specifically Alzheimer's (the most common form of dementia), revealed that the disease is surprisingly common, a leading cause of death, and can be incubating for as long as 25 years before one becomes symptomatic. This is quite alarming to me as a 43-year-old. In the United States for instance, it's estimated that 50 percent of people aged 85 have it. Australian estimates are similar. In fact, the 2018 causes of death data released by the Australian Bureau of Statistics reported that cause of death by heart disease decreased by 22.4 percent since 2009, while dementia rates increased by 68.6 percent in the same period. Dementia is now the leading cause of death in Australian women and the second leading cause of death in men, following heart disease.

Imagine being told that in around 25 years you'd have a 50 percent chance that you'd sustain a debilitating head injury in a car accident, which would result in significant memory impairment and an inability to live independently. How might you prepare to avoid such a situation? Would you engage in a defensive driving course? Consider buying a Volvo? Or even refrain from driving at all?

Given we know about the Alzheimer's disease incubation period, and how common it is, and how it impacts memory and independent living, what might we do to avoid such a situation? Batten down the hatches as if you were avoiding a car crash? Quite the opposite in fact. The best research on prevention of cognitive decline and dementia (including Alzheimer's) points to long term lifestyle enrichment. Connection with others, novelty, passion, purpose; an enriched life is more protective and resilient than a restricted one.

There's no time like the present to build one's reserves and I personally engage in the recommendations outlined in this book. I like to think like entrepreneur and physician, Dr. Peter Diamandis, who recommends adopting a longevity mindset. He believes it's perfectly reasonable for us to consider the age of 100 as the new 60. A longevity mindset is about being proactive about seeking out and engaging with those activities that can help you live a longer and healthy life.

Each of the strategies outlined in this book are intended to help you protect and enhance your cognitive abilities and maintain flexibility in thinking. Not every modality will suit all of you. We're all different and resonate with different things. There's no one-size-fits-all approach. For some it will be physical activities and meditation. Others will prefer creative endeavors or online brain training. You might like to learn a language, or travel, might appeal.

I've really just scratched the surface with the specific modalities addressed here as a catalyst to stimulate your own journey. I'd love to hear how this book may have served as a catalyst for you to create a flourishing life, so please feel free to contact me at **andrew@neuaudio.com.au**.

Purpose

It's important to remember that each of these methods can only be effective when sustained over the long term. For this to occur, they need to resonate or be of interest to you. Science tells us it pays to have a mission or purpose and a goal-setting strategy to fulfil a regular task. A degree of self-awareness can be helpful here.

If you were to wave a magic wand and suddenly your brain increased its potential by 50 percent, what would you wish for? For me, words would come to me more swiftly and readily, which would help me in my clinical work, presentations, and social life.

Earlier this year I was somewhat derailed by the untimely death of my sister; many of the good habits I had established simply went out the window. You may have had similar experiences where you've been firing on all cylinders and then something disrupts that. No matter your stage of life—be it mid-career or retirement—having self-awareness, a sense of purpose and a goal-setting strategy can be immensely powerful to help you achieve your ideals. It's so powerful that I've included extensive material on this later in this book.

Many of my patients have found me via my seminars either directly or by being referred by someone who attended. This has afforded me a patient group that is generally proactive about their health and open to new insights.

Our journey together begins with an introductory phone or Zoom call ahead of their initial appointment so that I can get to know them, their issues, and to learn a little about how their hearing deficits affect their lifestyle. A full assessment follows, which typically takes around an hour and a half. Follow-up appointments ensure they're coping well with the device and allow for any necessary adjustments.

I like to see my patients once every six months to make sure they're able to wear their devices full-time and to ensure they're appropriately adjusted. So over the years we work together, I get to know my patients well and it's clear to me that those who wear their devices consistently experience benefits beyond simply being able to follow conversation at a cocktail party. I've observed that full-time wearers seem to maintain their faculties better than the minority who leave their devices in the top drawer.

Time with my patients is essential to the understanding that wearing their hearing aids has a major impact on their lives and health. This is quite a different dynamic to what one might have with a GP, where in Australia, the average appointment time is just under 15 minutes, and around 17 minutes in the United States. There's little time in these circumstances to deal with anything other than diagnosing and prescribing.

I also take great pleasure in mentoring my own clinical staff and helping other independent clinicians to adopt a similar philosophy to the way they practice. My goal is to spread best practices as wide as I possibly can while helping talented clinicians do the same.

Writing *Your Resilient Brain* was a way to further my goal of providing suggestions that will help all my patients achieve optimum health and psychological flourishing. I'm not a psychologist, nutritionist, exercise physiologist, medical doctor, or neurologist, just an avid researcher and unapologetic geek. When I find useful stuff, I just want to share it.

This book is presented in two parts. Part 1: A Case for Connection and Part 2: Caring for Cognition. In the first part, I outline importance of human connection, of meaning and purpose with reference to how the practice of meditation can assist in these endeavors. The second part outlines additional, scientifically backed specific methods for protecting and enhancing cognitive health.

If you're interested in learning more about the connection between hearing and cognitive decline, you may be interested in my first book,

Hearing & Brain Health or book in for a free live seminar via **https://neuaudio.com.au/** or enroll on our complimentary, online Hearing & Brain Health Academy at **https://neuaudio.link/brainhealth**

PART 1

A Case For Connection

CHAPTER 1

Put your ears in, darl

*Three retirees with untreated
hearing loss are playing golf.
One remarked, "Windy, isn't it?"
"No," said the second man, "it's Thursday."
The third man said,
"So am I. Let's have a beer."*

Why it's imperative to wear your hearing devices full time

Traditionally, hearing aids have been a bit of a thorny subject; their popularity could be seen as akin to downing a spoon of castor oil. People associate them with getting old. Vanity has played its part as well—who wants clunky great beige bananas skirting their ears? Never mind that those clunky bananas have morphed into refined, barely detectible devices with Bluetooth capability that offer interactivity with your smartphone and TV, the stigma still prevents people from attending to the delicate organs that are vital for a happy interaction with all that life offers.

Research shows that people often put up with hearing loss for between 7-10 years before they take action. Those who do finally fess up and attend an audiologist, go to the expense of purchasing a pair of aids yet they neglect to wear them.

Hearing aids must be worn for between 12-16 hours a day, not just within a group or social situation. If I had a dollar for every person I've encountered over my 20-year career who didn't wear their hearing aids properly, I'd be able to buy an island and retreat into a quiet life in nature. Do you hear me?

Anyone who's had their hearing treated at my practice will tell you I'm fanatical (in the nicest possible way) about full-time hearing aid use, and the result is that my clients have an over 90 percent compliance rate. It's simply the best advice I can give any hearing-device owner. Apart from bathing, swimming, and sleeping, the more your devices are in, the more beneficial they'll be in the immediate and long term.

Nevertheless, a surprisingly high number of people who own hearing aids don't wear them adequately. In a major study of 13,591 Australian hearing aid owners (published 2015), Dr. Anthony Hogan found that approximately one third don't wear their devices at all or for less than two hours a day. One third wears them only 2-12 hours per day, and the remaining third wears them 12-plus hours a day. Anecdotal evidence and my own direct experience would suggest similar trends occur worldwide. There are three trends that show up regularly in my practice:

1. **Hearing aid owners simply weren't told to wear them every waking hour.**

Not a week goes by that I don't explain the benefits of full-time use to someone who has purchased their hearing aids elsewhere. It's almost as if they were hearing this advice for the first time. Perhaps the audiologist who fitted the devices was short on time or wasn't educated regarding the benefits of full-time use.

The most important thing your audiologist can do for you is advise, monitor, and wholeheartedly encourage your full-time use. I estimate that around 50 percent of my clinical time is in some way related to ensuring the conditions are such that my patients actually wear their devices. One of the great features of modern hearing aids is that their usage can be monitored at in-clinic appointments by your audiologist because databases are built into all devices.

2. The acclimatization period was incomplete.

When we finally do address our hearing deficits (be it a delay of three or 30 years) and have hearing aids fitted, there's a lot to get used to. It's an adaptive process. Like a muscle that hasn't been exercised, the neural pathways take time to strengthen.

The brain also needs to re-learn to filter the useful sounds from those that are not. This filter re-setting simply takes time. For most people, 12-16 hours of use a day over 7-10 days at conservative settings does the trick, and sometimes further adjustment is needed. It's a personalized process depending on the degree of loss, how long the hearing loss has been around, personal sound preferences, and volume tolerance. The early stages are the most challenging, but they are a crucial aspect of success. With time and patience, everything tends to get better and feel more natural.

3. Devices were uncomfortable for full-time use.

If they're not comfortable, they simply won't be worn the way they need to be. In experienced hands, the physical fit can be improved substantially. Volume and noise-reduction settings can also be adjusted in most cases, as long as the hearing device is sophisticated enough to allow fine adjustments.

Sometimes people are concerned about the look of the device. This is less of an issue these days because they are much more subtle and cosmetically pleasing.

What's the point of wearing my hearing aids full-time?

Hearing is completely different to vision, so hearing aids should not be worn only for conversation the way reading glasses are used sporadically for reading. The full benefits and value of hearing aids can only happen with full-time use.

The optic nerves are the only parts of our brains that protrude beyond our skulls, making them a direct brain interface. The process of seeing is essentially switched off the moment we close our eyes.

On the other hand, hearing happens in the brain beyond our ears. These processes are 'switched on' 24/7—even during sleep. The role of our peripheral hearing system (our ears) is to convert sound (rapid changes in air pressure) into electrical impulses which are, put simply, a language of the brain. From the ear, these impulses are sent to the hearing centers in the brain.

The most common forms of hearing loss occur at the point where the energy from sound (those rapid changes in air pressure) are converted to electrical impulses, which happens at the nerve endings or hair cells. We only hear sounds when these impulses are generated by the ear for the brain to process. Then an elaborate set of crossover processes happens between hearing centers on both sides of the brain so that we can focus on what we want to hear and filter out what we don't.

Hearing loss presents a barrier or a hurdle for sound stimulation to reach the brain's hearing centers, and has a rather dramatic impact on our ability to focus on what we're wanting to listen to. When only part of the day is amplified by hearing devices, it's hard for the brain to know which sounds are helpful and which aren't. For instance, the sounds of the clock ticking or the whirring of the refrigerator motor are always there, but having our hearing focused on them serves no regular or useful purpose. Ordinarily, you only really hear them when you listen out for them.

If you're wearing hearing devices for the first time, the brain needs to re-learn where to apply the filters on helpful versus unhelpful sounds. Although the process takes time, it occurs far more quickly when all the listening you're doing occurs through the devices. Inevitable changes to the way you hear your own voice also become more natural when you wear your devices full-time.

Don't fall for the hearing myth

Another benefit of full-time use is the reduced risk of falls. Studies show that untreated hearing loss, even at mild levels, results in a 300 percent increased risk of falls for 40-69-year-olds. Researchers cite two main reasons; the first being environmental awareness. With untreated hearing loss, you're less likely to hear things that may trip you up such as the sound of your feet on steps, which could cause you to fall, or that bike or scooter whizzing past when you're out for a walk. The second reason is that the sheer mental resources it takes to compensate for hearing loss leaves less attention for steadiness and balance.

Falls account for 25 percent of all hospital admissions and 40 percent of all nursing home admissions; 40 percent of those admitted do not return to independent living and 25 percent pass away within a year. As alarming as these statistics are, they're an underestimation because many falls go unreported. Separate to this, a major cause of falls in the elderly is when they get up to answer the phone. Some of the latest hearing aids integrate with mobile phones and are handsfree, so there's no need for elderly people to rush to answer the phone. Full-time hearing aid use helps nullify the risk of falls by improving environmental awareness.

Today's hearing aids are modern marvels with apps and Bluetooth and the ability to make them comfortable in every way, but it's vital to wear them for 12–16 hours per day. If comfort is an issue, speak to your audiologist.

The main reason I ask patients to come in for a six-monthly review appointment is to ensure they're wearing their devices full-time. It's also prudent to check hearing levels annually or check that the devices are tuned optimally.

Breaking the noise barrier

A common objection I hear about full-time use of hearing devices is that they actually increase the levels of background noise. This is true of many older style devices, however, advances in neuroscience have designed hearing aids that help overcome those extraneous sounds.

A high degree of 'teamwork' occurs between the ears, which assists in reducing the perception of background noise. We call this binaural (meaning both ears) ability. When the hearing system is damaged, we lose much of our binaural ability.

Many of the new-age hearing aids have a function called binaural beamforming, which allows the microphones to work together as a team, supplementing this impaired ability. This means a person is 30 percent more able to understand speech in background noise with binaural beaming than with hearing aids that don't have that capability. Several studies have shown that binaural beamforming technology can give wearers an advantage over people with normal hearing, provided their hearing loss is in the mild to moderate range.

The other aspect of urgency with regard to the use of binaural devices is borne out in a recently published study, July 2021 (*Alzheimer's & Dementia: The Journal of the Alzheimer's Association*). Researchers at University of Oxford's Nuffield Department of Population Health investigated the link between Alzheimer's disease and hearing loss in the largest study of its kind. A group of 82,000 women and men aged 60-plus were tested for 11 years for struggling to hear speech-in-noise (inability to hear in noisy situations). The study demonstrated that "insufficient" and "poor" speech-in-noise hearing were associated with a 61 percent and 91 percent increased risk of developing dementia, compared to normal speech-in-noise hearing, respectively.

The two sides of hearing devices

The brain has two hemispheres that are divided by a thick band of around 250 million nerve fibers (corpus callosum), which is the communication vehicle between the two sides. Generally speaking, the right side of the brain controls the left side of the body and vice-versa.

It's like that for hearing as well. When our hearing systems are working normally, around 80 percent of everything we hear goes to the opposite side of the brain. An elaborate feedback system sends the sounds to nerve endings at the opposite ear to give us the ability to focus on what we want to hear and separate out what we don't.

While conventional directional microphones have significantly improved the signal-to-noise ratio—the balance between sounds you want to hear vs sounds that you don't—it's simply not enough, so hearing someone speak in the presence of a lot of background noise is still difficult. Fortunately, several manufacturers utilize binaural beamforming technology. I only recommend devices with binaural function because of the significantly increased benefits for communication and cognition.

Untreated hearing loss requires increased listening effort, which increases cognitive load, or strain on the brain. There are specific brainwave patterns for listening effort that can be picked up by EEG electrodes on the skull; studies have shown that binaural beamforming devices require less listening effort to understand speech in noisy situations. Studies have also shown that memory recall for conversations in background noise is also better with binaural beamforming devices, largely due to reduced cognitive load.

Binaural beamforming alone is not sufficient to deliver such benefits; literally thousands of adjustments can be made by the audiologist to match the technology correctly to the wearer. We also make sure that the model and look of the device is appropriate for the wearer and their lifestyle. And remember, it's crucial that the devices are worn consistently—at least 12 hours per day. That way you're giving your brain the opportunity to learn to filter out all those unwanted sounds.

CHAPTER 2

Social interaction

Core Benefits: Social benefits and mood enhancement

Effective communication is central to maintaining quality relationships. Children who can't hear have difficulty developing speech. By nature, we're social creatures and we use all the senses to interact with each other, however, our primary way of interacting is through our hearing.

Loss of hearing affects everything including physical, spiritual, and mental wellbeing. As an audiologist it's a no brainer that I deal with social interaction as a vital element of hearing. Certainly, preserving human connection underpins everything I do in my clinics and patient education programs.

The primary challenge facing hearing impaired people is difficulty hearing in social situations. Relationships, too, are affected and often the loved ones of those with hearing loss are equally or more impacted by the condition. For a heart-to-heart conversation to work, two people need to hear each other. I've seen patients who require separate television rooms because one partner cannot hear at a level that is comfortable for the other.

When it all gets too hard, people with hearing loss may stop going to the movies because they can't hear the dialogue, or they stay away from shopping malls and restaurants because of the overwhelming background noise that makes it impossible to hear what someone is saying. The withdrawal from and avoidance of those environments can have terrible consequences.

Psychologists talk about the long-term psychological impacts of social isolation, and decades of research indicates that it's a risk factor for developing anxiety, depression, heart disease and, ultimately, having a reduced quality of life and longevity.

In my Hearing and Brain Health Seminars I stress that one of the main reasons we want to treat hearing loss is to maintain social connection. The Grant and Glueck study—an ongoing, 80 year-long study of adult development out of Harvard University— demonstrates that quality relationships keep us happier and healthier long-term above any other factor.

In one study, researchers examined vast amounts of medical records and hundreds of interviews and questionnaires and found a strong correlation between happy marriages and the experience of pain, whereby people in their eighties who were in happy marriages reported that when they suffered pain their mood didn't suffer. Also, that people who were the most satisfied in their relationships at age 50 were the healthiest at age 80, and the state of people's relationships when they were age 50 was a better predictor of physical health than cholesterol levels.

Director of the study, psychiatrist Robert Waldinger commented that people who maintained good relationships lived happier and longer whereas loners often died earlier. He said that loneliness has a physical effect that is as powerful as smoking or alcoholism.

In a longitudinal study of ageing undertaken between 2004-2012 in the United Kingdom, they surveyed 6,500 people aged 52 and over. They discovered that social isolation was correlated with higher mortality, and that limited contact with family, friends and community groups was a predictor of illness and earlier death. This was regardless of whether the individuals felt lonely.

The experience of dealing with the COVID-19 pandemic also shines a light on the potentially devastating impact of social isolation. One study published in scientific journal *PLOS One*, investigated the acute mental health responses of Australian adults during the pandemic. More than 5,000 adults were questioned by investigators from the University of New South Wales during the peak of the pandemic and the initial lockdown. The result was that 78 percent of respondents reported their mental health had worsened since the outbreak. Accompanying the fear that they and their loved ones might contract the disease, was loneliness and the uncertainty of what was to come. Rates of depression, anxiety and stress levels skyrocketed by between 50-65 percent.

Place hearing impediments on top of that and the world becomes very contracted. You might be able to see people on Zoom, but you may not be able to have a conversation that doesn't involve disengagement, frustration and/or raised voices.

The Australian Institute of Health and Welfare (AIHW) cites risk factors for social isolation and loneliness as being hearing loss, disconnection from community, relationship breakups, mental illness, and living alone. According to AIHW and Relationships Australia data, social isolation is associated with mental illness, emotional distress, suicide, the development of dementia, premature death, poor health behaviors, smoking, physical inactivity, poor sleep, and biological effects, including high blood pressure and poorer immune function.

Psychologist Susan Pinker wrote a fascinating book about the importance of social interaction on wellbeing and longevity called, *The Village Effect*. It demonstrates how crucial it is to experience face-to-face contact in relation to learning, happiness, resilience, and longevity. In this book she uses the example of the blue zones that I frequently talk about in my seminars.

Blue zones are regions in the world where people typically live healthier and longer than average—often over a century. The blue zones include Okinawa in Japan, Sardinia in Italy, Nicoya in Costa Rica, Ikaria in Greece, and Loma Linda in California. One difference they discovered in Sardinia was that men tended to have equal life expectancy to women whereas in the other blue zones, and here in the West, women outlive men by around eight years. The researchers concluded that the key differentiator was that Sardinian men placed equal importance to women on nurturing quality relationships.

Being alone is not the same as loneliness. After a long day at work or a full-on time with the family, one can crave some quiet time. We all need a modicum of solitude; time to reflect, wind down, chill out, time to remember who you are. This is a very different circumstance to feeling lonely and isolated where you generally have very little contact with others and feel perhaps unloved or disconnected from people.

The 20th and 21st centuries have seen us become more globally connected than ever. But this kind of connection does not necessarily mean one feels *connected*. What may add to a sense of loneliness is the way we use social media. It has become de rigueur to communicate electronically with the people we care about. Via social media, we announce to the world what we ate for breakfast, which café we're in, or send a text to say hi, but this kind of communication does not replace the direct eye contact, the face-to-face, the quality of actually being in someone's presence, which humans need on a biological and emotional level. I wonder, could we lose the ability to have relationships that have depth and strength because rather than talking to someone, we text them.

"After my recent brush with voicelessness, I thought I'd share with you a few thoughts about speech. Don't take it lightly my friends. If music is the pathway to the heart as Voltaire suggested, then speech is the pathway to other people. Live in silence and you live alone."

~Henry Bromell

CHAPTER 3

The greatest love

Core Benefits: Enhanced mental, spiritual and physical health

Living in a state of gratitude can have a huge impact on your life and health. On a chemical and physical level, the expression of gratitude causes the brain to release surges of neurotransmitters dopamine and serotonin, which takes immediate effect and elevates us to a cheerier state. These neurotransmitters play a vital role in various abilities such as experiencing pleasure and the joys of reward, as well as assisting with regulating the body's physical movements.

Emotional health

Studies conducted across the past decade have shown that people who live in a state of conscious appreciation, tend to be happier and less depressed. It's also been shown to be beneficial for people who struggle with mental health issues.

A study was conducted on mostly college students (293 adults) who suffered from clinical depression and anxiety and sought counselling services at their university. Participants were randomly placed into three groups which each received counselling. The first group was instructed to write one letter of gratitude to someone each week for three weeks. The second group was asked to write about their deepest thoughts and feelings about negative experiences. The third group did no writing activity.

The group who wrote letters of gratitude reported significantly better mental health when measured at four then 12 weeks after the end of the writing exercise. So, it would seem that practicing gratitude in addition to psychological counselling enhances the benefit.

Velcro and Teflon

Another aspect of being consciously grateful is that it distracts us and dislodges our grip on negative emotions, providing a new perspective. Once you develop a regular practice, a new perspective is wired into the brain.

According to psychologist Rick Hanson, the brain

has a negative bias. He says that the mind is like Velcro for negative experiences and Teflon for positive ones. If something embarrassing happens, we may dwell on it for weeks or more. It overwhelms us far more than a positive experience, and with every experience, our brain's neural pathways are rewritten.

Developing that negative bias was an early survival instinct, whereby our earliest ancestors needed to be on constant alert for environmental dangers. However, the latest neuroscience findings show us that negativity bias can be modified because our brains are plastic. Several activities actually thicken the insula, which is the part of the brain that, among other things, senses the internal state of the body, and our feelings.

The Insula interacts closely with the prefrontal cortex and the amygdala. You may recall these structures are associated with the extent to which our brains are resilient to adversity. With reference to the 1986 Nun study on Alzheimer's mentioned in the introduction; at risk of oversimplification, I speculate that the Nun's found to have resilient brains had developed capacities akin to Velcro for the positive and Teflon for the negative.

The research demonstrates that when you're doing focused activities such as meditation, or yoga or practicing gratitude, the insula becomes thicker because the neurons are making more connections, so people become more in touch with themselves and more empathetic to others.

A heartfelt practice

When practiced daily, gratefulness can have an impact on our physical health. Take heart attacks for instance. University of Connecticut researchers studied people who'd had one heart attack. Those who saw some worth in the illness such as a greater appreciation in the value of their life, had a significantly lower risk of another heart attack.

Professor of Psychology, UC Davis, Dr. Robert Emmons conducted several studies on the effects of gratitude. His findings show that it can strengthen the immune system, enhance brain power and quality of sleep, reduce pain, and improve digestion.

How to develop a daily gratitude practice

Challenging events happen all the time. People get sick, they die, there's grief, pain, war, pandemics, and arguments. This is life. We can view life as a series of disasters or we can 'wire in' a state of acceptance, and appreciation of the abundance we already have.

A daily, conscious practice of gratitude can rewrite our neural pathways and create a lasting effect on the way we feel. Create a simple gratitude journal and list around 10 things you're grateful for each day. Strengthening these neural pathways makes us more permanently grateful and forward-looking. Feeling the emotion of gratitude as you write each point will further embed the change. Even easier, simply commit genuinely to starting each day with a grateful heart.

Gratitude doesn't mean you're merely appreciative of something that happens now and then. It's about appreciating every moment like it's your last because we never know when that moment will be. Motivation guru Tony Robbins describes people with this mindset as having an 'attitude of gratitude'.

If we're always looking towards that next fix—I'll be happy when I have enough money, a better house, when I have the right golf clubs—how can we possibly see the value in the life we currently have?

The thing that money can't buy is another moment.

The following link is to a magnificent audio piece by Benedictine monk Brother David Steindl-Rast, who spent much of his life touring the world, lecturing on grateful living. Go to gratefulness.org and click on 'Practice' then 'A Grateful Day'.

"...it is your mind, rather than circumstances themselves that determines the quality of your life. The mind is the basis of everything you experience."

~Sam Harris

CHAPTER 4

Stress relief

Core Benefit: Maintain hearing health and reduce the risk of illness

There are two kinds of stress: good stress, which motivates you to get out of bed every day; and negative stress, which is the modern disease. Negative stress is a root cause of many ill-health conditions, including hearing.

When we encounter a stressor, our body releases stress hormones to provide a burst of energy or strength. Our blood vessels constrict and divert more oxygen to the muscles, which increases your strength to take action. It also raises blood pressure, and frequent or chronic stress can make your heart work too hard over long periods, which can cause oxidative damage and inflammation.

Oxidative stress can damage cells, which may eventually weaken the immune system and lead to a range of diseases. It's also considered to be the primary mechanism behind impaired nerve endings that results in sensorineural hearing loss—the most common form of hearing loss.

Constant stress stops the body receiving that clear signal to return to normal. Eventually it can lead to serious health problems such as heart disease, high blood pressure, diabetes and other illnesses, all of which can affect your hearing.

One side effect of daily stress and the overproduction of adrenaline is the reduction of blood flow throughout the body, including the ears. The hair cells in the inner ear rely on constant blood flow for delivery of oxygen and nutrients. Without it, those fragile hair cells can become damaged. Sometimes permanently.

The following information on meditation can help you reduce stress and bring harmony to your daily lives.

MEDITATION

Core Benefits: Stress reduction and cognitive enhancement

"Meditation takes us from survival to creation; from separation to connection; from imbalance to balance; from emergency mode to growth-and-repair mode; and from the limiting emotions of fear, anger, and sadness to the expansive emotions of joy, freedom, and love."

~Dr. Joe Dispenza.

Some of you might feel uncomfortable with the idea of meditation. Some might think it's a new-age fad. However, my extensive research into the science of meditation has demonstrated time and time again that the benefits of the practice are consistently substantial. Meditation allows us to access states of peak performance and fulfilment. Its potential for stress reduction is undeniable and as you'll learn, it can even create beneficial changes to brain structure.

Tim Ferris is an American entrepreneur, author, investor, and lifestyle guru. He became an advocate for the practice of meditation after writing *Tools of Titans: The Tactics, Routines, and Habits of Billionaires, Icons, and World-Class Performers*. The book is based on his interviews with more than 200 people who are at their top of their respective fields; this includes celebrities, athletes, and scientists. One habit that was consistently common to the Titans he interviewed was the practice of meditation.

In a similar book, *Game Changers: What Leaders, Innovators and Mavericks Do to Win at Life*, Dave Asprey mirrors Tim Ferris' findings. He reports that of the 450 experts that inspired the book, the practice of meditation was their most consistently reported habit.

Ferris says that more than 80 percent of the world-class performers he interviewed, independent of their specialty, used meditation to achieve better results with less stress. Many were using the practice to recover from the feeling of 'being in the trenches' throughout the day. He summed up with a quote by Abraham Lincoln: "Give me six hours to chop down a tree and I'll spend the first four sharpening the axe."

In Tim's words, "Meditation simply helps you channel drive toward the few things that matter, rather than every moving target and imaginary opponent that pops up."

Another proponent of meditation is Yuval Harari, a professor in the Department of History at the Hebrew University of Jerusalem, and a best-selling author. His books are about what makes us uniquely human. He writes about our capacity for communication and the challenge that artificial intelligence is likely to present in the near future. Harari describes meditation as the best tool to develop psychological flexibility and resilience.

Harari meditates for two hours a day and attends at least one three-to-six-week meditation retreat each year. He claims that there's no way he'd be able to do the work without having developed the mental clarity, concentration and focus that meditation brings.

For me, the most tangible benefit I get from the practice relates to what is known as the 'default mode network', a brain network associated with mind wandering and self-related thinking. Overactivity in the default mode network has been shown to be related to unhappiness and cognitive fatigue.

A major study of 5000 people found that participants who were thinking about something other than the activity they were doing, were caught up in their default mode network for at least half of the time. It also found that people were most happy when they were thinking about what they were actually doing at that point in time, even happier than when their mind was wandering on positive thoughts.

The researchers said, "A human mind is a wandering mind, and a wandering mind is an unhappy mind." It's well documented that the practice of meditation is associated with reduced activity in the default mode network. In other words, the voice inside one's head, that inner critic tends to quieten; I've personally found that to be the most obvious benefit. When I meditate, I simply get more done. When my meditation practice has lapsed for a time, my mind wanders more and focused attention becomes more difficult.

Meditation was once primarily a faith-based practice, perhaps reserved for monks in temples and caves. The 20th century saw the various practices become increasingly popular and the benefits are now backed by rigorous scientific enquiry. One well studied modality is Transcendental Meditation

(TM) a simple technique that has profound effects. More than 600 studies have been conducted into TM. One study funded by the National Institutes of Health found that African-Americans with heart disease who regularly practiced TM had a 48 percent reduced risk of death, heart attack and stroke.

The link between stress and cardiovascular disease (CVD) is well defined and so unsurprising given the ability of TM to reduce the long-lasting effects of stress, it's been found to be useful in the prevention and treatment of CVD. It's also proven to be effective in treating soldiers with PTSD. Children who meditate twice a day sleep better, are more creative thinkers and achieve better academically. They're healthier, have higher self-esteem and experience significant reductions in stress, anxiety and depressive symptoms.

If I could recommend one habit to anyone I care about, it would be to develop the habit of meditating. My preferred practice is mindfulness-based. Mindfulness meditation gained popularity in the Western world in part because like TM it doesn't require any specific religious faith, and there's a lot of scientific evidence for the various benefits.

Practicing meditation may play a role in hearing loss prevention, improving the hearing centers in the brain, and reduces tinnitus (ringing in the ears) disturbance.

Meditation and hearing health

If you suffer from tinnitus, meditation can improve your ability to selectively switch attention away from the sounds throughout your day. During meditation sessions, it can be helpful to pay attention to the tinnitus sound, so you can start to associate it with the positive experience of relaxation and calm. This new, more peaceful association may slowly replace the old disturbing and stressful one. Also, you might consider playing some relaxing sounds or music during meditation sessions if you find the tinnitus particularly distracting.

One of the main benefits of meditation relates to its strong potential to reduce stress. Stress is a primary exacerbator of tinnitus. Prolonged exposure to the fight or flight chemicals creates inflammation and can result in the deterioration of your health, which includes the delicate parts within the ears.

The overproduction of adrenaline can reduce

blood circulation in the inner ear. Not only can this cause hearing loss over time, in rare cases there can be sudden hearing loss when circulation stops completely. Meditation lowers the production of adrenaline and increases the flow of blood within the ears. That blood flow is essential to maintaining hearing health. Additionally, the stress response can result in oxidative stress, which is largely a result of an imbalance between free radicals and antioxidants.

Meditation, which reduces stress, also decreases these deteriorating health effects. According to research conducted by Sara Lazar, neuroscientist at the Massachusetts General Hospital, meditation goes a step further and can be beneficial to the primary hearing centers of the brain, particularly those located in the temporal lobe including the auditory cortex, the main area of the brain specific to hearing. According to a meta-analysis of several published studies, "Those who meditated have an increased thickness of grey matter in parts of the brain responsible for attention compared to those who do not meditate."

It's not just a boost in focus, meditating increases the way the brain codes and stores auditory information. Separate to the physiological benefits on the auditory system, meditation has been shown to increase the qualities of compassion and empathy in practitioners. Combined with attentional improvements, it follows that you may well become a better listener. How can that not be a good thing?

If you're wondering where to begin, it's worth trying out different methods to see how they suit you. I've tried several methods over the past five years and I have to say that the 'Waking Up' smartphone app by neuroscientist and philosopher Sam Harris is the most helpful and comprehensive way to get started that I've been able to find. It's a guided meditation, non-religious, based on science and easy to follow. I find it best to listen to after exercise. He has also written a book called *Waking Up*. For more information check out **www.wakingup.com**.

Floating away

Another practice I really love as an addition to my meditation is the sensory isolation of being in a flotation tank; it's like meditation on steroids. Every time I go for a 'float', it's like reaching that point on a holiday where you're completely relaxed.

Scientific research suggests that time spent floating in a sensory deprivation tank is beneficial to muscle relaxation, better sleep, decrease in pain, and decreased stress and anxiety. I can recommend the services of Beyond Rest; they have several float centers around Australia. Check out **beyondrest. com.au**.

Many people who are just starting meditation wonder whether they are doing it correctly. To counter this anxiety, I use a Muse headset. Muse is a research grade, portable EEG (electroencephalogram) worn like a small headband during meditation. It measures brainwaves and delivers biofeedback via a smartphone app to let you know if you're on track. For advanced meditators there's an additional app called Muse Monitor, which provides additional insights into progress. It measures the specific alpha, beta, delta, gamma and theta brainwaves. Check out choosemuse.com. Otherwise, you can just get on with meditating and know that even though you may not be able to still your mind or rid yourself of random thoughts, it is still working. Every time you come back to the meditation object, most commonly the breath, you're strengthening your attentional capabilities.

If you're interested in exploring the field of meditation further, I highly recommend the work of Dr. Joe Dispenza. He's written several books on the topic and has developed a range of online resources. He aims to demystify meditation by explaining the science behind the practice.

Getting to the heart of the matter

Have you had the experience of knowing something in your heart? There's a reason for that. It might surprise you to know that the heart contains around 40,000 neurons that can sense, feel, learn and remember, which is to say our heart also has neuroplasticity. So in a sense, the heart is part brain. The 'brain' aspect of our heart sends messages to the brain in the head about a whole range of things.

Research carried out in the 1990s showed that the brain/heart relationship is a two-way street; messages go from the brain to the heart to the brain, neurotransmitters and proteins, just like those in the brain that message the heart.

The experience of positive emotions such as compassion and caring takes place in the heart and serves to bring coherence to our heart's rhythm.

Research undertaken by the HeartMath Institute demonstrates that different emotional states create different patterns of heart activity and these in turn have distinct effects on cognitive and emotional function. The pattern of the heart's rhythm becomes measurably erratic and disordered when someone experiences negative emotions and stress. These more chaotic neural signals going from the heart to the brain can impede higher cognitive functions. Our memory and ability to think, reason and make good decisions may fly out the window because of it.

On the other hand, positive emotions that are communicated to the brain can enhance and facilitate cognitive function as well as reinforce positive feelings and emotional stability. The heart processes these emotions, which make the heart's rhythm more coherent and harmonious. These factors are objectively measurable and affect the entire body.

Through conscious effort, you can listen to what the intelligence of your heart tells you and by so doing, make clear, heartfelt, and harmonious decisions. Like any skill, this ability can be strengthened with practice, there are many heart centred meditative techniques supported by scientific enquiry that are focussed on this. According to the HeartMath institute, you can even learn to shift into this coherent state, which brings your mind and heart into harmonious alignment, sustaining positive emotions and mental clarity that affect how we feel, think and perceive the world.

For more information about the heart/brain connection go to **https://www.heartmath.org/**

CHAPTER 5

Meaning and purpose

Core Benefits: Enhanced emotional and physical health, and feeling deeply satisfied with your life

"Life is without meaning. You bring meaning to it. The meaning of life is whatever you ascribe it to be. Being alive is the meaning."

~Joseph Campbell

When you boil it all down, we only have now. The past is no longer available, nor is the future within our grasp. That means that *now* is the most important moment of your life. People who suffer from anxiety are worried about things that haven't happened; they live in fear of what *could* happen. So, the future is a threat. Excessively dwelling on the past can lead to depression. So, do we live in between the cracks in the life continuum? Or, do we fully embrace what life has to offer each moment?

Now for my next pithy question: what does the search for meaning and purpose have to do with our hearing and cognitive health? Our bodies and minds are a complete circuit. Everything is interconnected and living within one entity. Our emotions affect our physical wellbeing, and our wellbeing includes our ears and hearing.

It's been scientifically established that having purpose in life can reduce the risk of Alzheimer's disease and cognitive impairment. In 2010, two researchers, Dr. David Bennett and Dr. Pamela Boyle from the Rush Medical Centre in Chicago, published the following findings in the *Archives of General Psychiatry*.

- A study of 951 older people without dementia, sought to establish the degree to which they had a sense of purpose and goals. Researchers followed them for more than seven years to see if they developed cognitive impairment or Alzheimer's symptoms. The results showed that 155 out of the 951 participants (16.3%) developed Alzheimer's disease and the statistical analysis revealed that having greater purpose in life was associated with a substantially reduced risk of developing Alzheimer's disease. People with purpose were approximately 2.4 times more likely to remain free of Alzheimer's than someone with a low purpose-in-life score.

People with a high-level purpose-in-life score were also linked to lesser rates of mild cognitive impairment, slower rates of cognitive decline in old age, and increased longevity. This is probably because they were less stressed and experienced more positive emotions.

Lack of purpose can make you feel depressed, worthless, and disconnected from yourself and those around you. In other words, it's a downer, and being down can affect your stress levels (cortisol) and immune system.

The question then is, if you're feeling somewhat lost and in despair, how do you discover your life's purpose? Perhaps you're looking in the wrong place, hoping that something 'out there' in your environment will provide you with satisfaction.

How time flies when you're having fun

Have you ever been totally engrossed in your work, a sport, music or even a conversation with a dear friend where time seemed to stand still or slip away completely? This state of being lost in an activity is described by Hungarian-American psychologist Mihaly Csikszentmihályi as being in the 'flow' state, which is being completely immersed in an activity for its own sake.

"The ego falls away. Time flies. Every action, movement, and thought follows inevitably from the previous one, like playing jazz. Your whole being is involved, and you are using your skills to the utmost."

Flow is like the runner's high, that feeling of euphoria caused by the rush of neurotransmitters, endorphins and endocannabinoids that makes you to want to continue the run because you feel relaxed. Athletes call it being in the zone; a place where there's no pain or anxiety.

In a state of flow, you feel at your best and perform accordingly. Each moment flows seamlessly and effortlessly to the next. There's a sense of fluidity between mind and body as you're completely absorbed in the activity and your focus is deep. You're in a place that's beyond distraction where nothing else seems to matter.

Flow triggers an extraordinary chain of events in our

brains, which is highly pleasant and can help spark a profound sense of meaning. It can accelerate learning and bring more richness to your life and, in turn, to the lives of others.

The concept was recognized and named by Mihaly Csikszentmihályi in 1975 after he conducted one of the largest psychological surveys ever. In the 1970s he interviewed people across the world about the times in their lives when they felt they were at their peak and performed at their best.

He began with top performers in a range of fields including chess players, surgeons, dancers, and athletes. Then, to better understand the universality of such experiences, he moved on to people who performed more commonplace jobs such as farmers, sheep herders, assembly line workers, teenage motorcycle gang members and cleaners. Everyone he spoke to, independent of culture, class, gender, age, or level of professional attainment performed and felt in their prime when they were experiencing the state that he termed flow.

Those who experience it rate it as the most enjoyable feeling on the planet, and they tend to want more of it. Legendary Brazilian Formula One driver, the late Ayrton Senna described it like this:

"And so you touch this limit, something happens and you suddenly can go a little bit further. With your mind power, your determination, your instinct, and the experience as well, you can fly very high. And suddenly I realized that I was no longer driving the car consciously. I was driving it by a kind of instinct, only I was in a different dimension... I continuously go further and further learning about my own limitations, my body limitation, psychological limitations. It's a way of life for me."

Dr. Csikszentmihályi adopted the word 'flow' because it kept coming up when speaking with his subjects because many described the experience as feeling 'flowy'. His seminal book *Flow: The Psychology of Optimal Experience*, really set the stage for serious enquiry into this fascinating phenomenon.

Renowned psychologist, Abraham Maslow established the hierarchy of needs. At the bottom of the pyramid, he put basic needs like food and shelter. At the top resides self-actualization, or fulfilling your potential—highly pleasurable experiences that result in giving us a profound sense of meaning. This is flow.

Understanding the nature of flow

Mihaly Csikszentmihályi characterized nine component states of achieving flow:

1. Challenge-skill balance (the activity is quite challenging)

2. Merging of action and awareness (mind and body seem as one)

3. Clarity of goals (the mind does not have to think about what to do next)

4. Immediate and unambiguous feedback (enables adjustment to current demands)

5. Concentration on the task at hand (complete immersion and focus)

6. Paradox of control (activities are automatic and fluid yet carried out with purpose)

7. Transformation of time (it seems to either slow down or speed up)

8. Loss of self-consciousness (the voice in your head disappears)

9. An autotelic experience (an activity worth doing in its own right)

Over the past 15 years, neuroscientists have made exceptional progress in helping us better understand the neurochemistry and neurophysiology of the flow experience. Contemporary brain imaging technologies and techniques have allowed them to objectively measure what not so long ago could only be described as a subjective experience. As attention sharpens in flow, slower energy intensive conscious processing is substituted for faster energy efficient subconscious processing.

According to neuroscientist Arne Dietrich, when we are in a state of flow, "We're trading energy usually used for higher cognitive functions for heightened attention and awareness." To be completely immersed in the moment, there's no room for internal chatter so we experience what is called transient hypofrontality whereby the prefrontal cortex—the focused, thinking part of the brain—goes offline. Time becomes distorted because the part of the brain that helps keep track of time is shut down.

Brainwave patterns and neurochemistry are also altered during this state. In flow, our brainwaves slow right down from fast-moving beta waves, which are the predominant thinking patterns that we have during our waking hours, and take us into the midpoint between alpha and theta waves, which is a daydream, hypnotic-like state. This induces a neurochemical cocktail that heightens our performance, accelerates learning, and creates a pleasurable experience.

While we are in this state, the neurotransmitters norepinephrine, dopamine, anandamide, serotonin and endorphins are all released at the same time. Combined, they help sharpen reaction times, attention, pattern recognition and lateral thinking. Each of these neurotransmitters are also highly addictive. It feels so good we just want more of it, and this leads to the autotelic (doing an activity for its own sake) nature of the flow states.

I first encountered a detailed account of flow in an inspirational book called *Bold*, by Steven Kottler and Peter Diamandis. It's a book that then President Bill Clinton described as, "A visionary roadmap for people who believe they can change the world..." *Bold* was one of the few books that I could not put down. The chapter on flow was the most exciting to me. The authors talked about it as being a tool to help entrepreneurs become more productive and to find a deep sense of meaning in what they do. For instance, they cite Sir Richard Branson as stating that he is five times more productive in flow—and we know how successful he's been. In fact, subsequent scientific studies of people in flow have shown that motivation goes up 500 percent, creativity up 600-700 percent and learning rates accelerate 470 percent.

Steven Kottler wrote three more best-selling books about flow. The most recent, *The Art of Impossible*, is the most comprehensive. If you're interested in learning more about it, I highly recommend Kottler's work.

One of the most exciting points Kottler makes is that neuroscience indicates that the flow state is universal and accessible to everyone.

"We are all hardwired for the experience. This echoes Csikszentmihàlyi's finding in the 1970s that the state is experienced by both peak performers and those engaged in seemingly mundane work."

I tend to experience flow most noticeably when delivering live seminars. Public speaking is widely considered a flow-inducing activity. During a presentation, several factors are in play: high consequences (what if they don't like me, or they're not engaged in the content?), unpredictable outcomes, or novelty (every crowd and venue is different), pattern recognition (use of slide prompts to avoid reading notes) and the challenge/skills ratio (I want each one to be better than the last). Sometimes it seems like a two-hour live seminar is over in 10 minutes. In others it seems like I've been presenting for four hours. When they've gone particularly well, the associated elation lasts for days.

It's my firm belief that being in the flow state has helped me with my live presentations on several fronts. Firstly, I now really enjoy and look forward to giving them. For me they are an autotelic activity, which means they are worthwhile doing in their own right. Secondly, I believe I've become much better at giving them, which suggests there's been some accelerated learning at play. I had one of the first seminars I delivered filmed, and compared it to one that was filmed around 50 seminars and two years later. They were like chalk and cheese.

Over time I've derived a deep sense of meaning from giving these presentations. When I think back to the early days of my career and remember the lengths people with hearing loss go to in order to avoid taking action, it was very frustrating. I could only reach one person at a time to help them understand the benefits of dealing with their hearing issues. What has given me the most career fulfillment are the times where I've been able to educate people on a grander scale.

Flow is a state of peak performance that can result in you realizing your 'calling', because the activity puts you in that state, or it can lead you to understand the joy in every moment. This can be life-changing.

I know that my work is my calling; what I truly believe I was meant to do, so I go with the flow. I've lost count of the number of people that report that they now wear their hearing devices at least 12 hours per day as a result of attending a seminar. After being inspired to take action, marriages have been saved, people have returned to work, and memory and general energy levels have improved. Some patients state that attending my seminar was one of the best things they've ever done because it inspired them to correct their hearing loss, something they've generally been putting off for years. Also, it's made them think more broadly about the effect hearing loss has not only on their lives, but the lives of people they care about.

The secondary flow-on effect of the seminars is

that my previous book, *Hearing & Brain Health*, that I often give away, gets passed around a lot, and each event usually follows an invitation to speak to at least one community group or club. Other audiology practices also regularly invite me to present on behalf of their clinics, and I have plans to speak internationally. I'm now privileged to be in a position to mentor other clinicians to give these kinds of presentations to help spread these important messages. This is all because I have been in a state of flow and on my path.

Consider something that you'd like to strive for, or things that have given you a sense of meaning in the past. Could it be ensuring that your family is happy and well cared for, adding value to the world through your work, creating inspiring art, helping people through volunteering, exploring the world, learning new things or improving yourself every day? Were you lost in that delightful flow zone?

For most of us, the flow state is fleeting, unpredictable and sporadic, but it needn't be. The practice of meditation is an ideal primer to achieve a flow state. In fact, there's some debate as to whether flow is a form of meditation or indeed whether experienced meditators are indeed entering a flow state. Nevertheless, neuroscience suggests there are significant parallels between meditation and flow.

A part of the brain that is particularly active during flow is the caudate nucleus. The caudate is involved with control of voluntary movement as well as being an important element of the brain's learning and memory system. Studies have shown that meditation improves the size and structure of this part of the brain, priming it to achieve a state of flow. Another more immediately recognizable benefit of meditation is that it helps you to be in the present. Flow occurs when our minds are focused on the now.

Living for now because today is all we have

"Stop acting as if life is a rehearsal. Live this day as if it were your last. The past is gone. The future is not guaranteed."

~Wayne Dyer

The mindfulness concept can help you stay focused on the present. Being mindful is to live in the moment and be fully in touch with reality, which includes your mind, emotions, body, and the outside world. Adopting and practicing this will give you greater insights into yourself and others. Changing your mode of operating takes persistence, especially if you're a particularly anxious person. With mindfulness meditation, most commonly you just sit quietly and follow your breath. When your mind wanders, you bring your focus back to the breath. The powerful point is the realization that you're lost in thought, noticing this and repeatedly coming back to the present moment strengthens one's capacity to be in the now.

Another important element that triggers flow is the challenge/skills ratio. Numerous studies indicate that when the challenge is around four percent above your current skill set, flow is often induced—enough to make you stretch but not enough to make you snap. According to Csikszentmihályi:

"The best moments in our lives are not the passive, receptive, relaxing times, the best moments usually occur if a person's body or mind is stretched to its limits in a voluntary effort to accomplish something difficult and worthwhile."

Flow lifts us out of the mundane and frequently gives us a sense of purpose. In fact, Csikszentmihàlyi's primary purpose for conducting the research was that he was trying to define the meaning of life after suffering the traumas of WW2 as a child. He became interested in discovering what contributes to a life that is worth living.

That's an important question that dogs many of us throughout our lives. We might feel trapped by circumstances that are less than optimum in our minds—the job is boring, the relationship lacks luster, our friends are not what we hoped; it's all exhausting. But what if we reframed all of that and found the joy in each activity or relationship?

As I write this, we're in another lockdown because of the COVID-19 pandemic. I could bemoan the fact and become mired in the sadness and isolation, the loss of income, restricted travel, uncertainty etcetera. I could heighten those feelings by focusing on them, or I could find the gift—perhaps that I have this opportunity to find new ways to add value, complete this book, connect with others in a new way.

In a 2015 interview, Csikszentmihályi said that if you want your life to have meaning, you have to give it one yourself. He says that for some people, meaning comes from the beauty of nature, the cosmos and/ or the variety and complexity of life itself.

"But the most sustaining meaning comes from what you yourself contribute to the world—by the love you give, the strength you provide, the beauty you create."

Another great thinker in the field was Austrian psychiatrist Dr. Victor Frankl. His book, *Man's Search for Meaning,* is a masterpiece that was declared to be one of the 10 most influential books in the United States. By the time he died in 1997, it had been translated into 24 languages and had sold over 16 million copies.

During WW2, Frankl was imprisoned in Theresien-stadt concentration camp, then Auschwitz. Most of his family were killed In the camps. In *Man's Search for Meaning,* he records his experiences as a prisoner and what he observed in others; their psychological reactions of shock, then apathy as they absorbed their situation, leading to deperson-alization, moral deformity, bitterness, and ultimately disillusionment if the person managed to survive.

Frankl concluded that a prisoner's psychological reactions were not solely the result of what was happening to them, but there was some freedom to choose what to think about life, even during extreme suffering. The strength of their spiritual self, relied on having hope. He observed that once a prisoner lost hope, they were doomed.

According to Frankl, the way a prisoner imagined their future also affected their longevity. He believed that the meaning of life is found in every moment, and that life never ceases to have meaning, even in suffering and death. Something to ponder deeply— is your glass half full or half empty?

The search for meaning can end here. You can decide if it lies in what you do, who you are, the difference you make to other's lives, how much you love yourself, how much you appreciate every moment, or in any and all of the above and more. Regardless of what you believe, it's hard to function optimally if we don't have reasonable health and wellbeing, and you cannot separate what takes place between the ears, from the ears.

Neurons that fire together wire together

There's a network in our brains called the reticular activating system (RAS), which is essentially a bundle of nerves in the brainstem that filter out unnecessary information so you can focus on what's important to you. The function of the RAS is demonstrated when you have a particular goal in mind. For instance, it's like if you start thinking seriously about buying a particular car and then suddenly you start seeing that same car at every turn. Do you recall the Teflon and Velcro analogy in the gratitude section? The RAS can be trained to be like Velcro for the things you want in life, and Teflon for those less important aspects.

It will also filter the world according to your beliefs and you'll generally see things that validate those beliefs. This is tied up with the power of intention, which means that focusing with intent on your goals may bring the people, information and opportunities that help you achieve them. 'Like attracts like' is the law of attraction.

However, there is a catch. The most crucial beliefs we have about ourselves, our deep internal belief system, is laid down in-utero where we begin to absorb the love and stresses of our parents' world. The process of embedding our beliefs continues until around age seven and they affect every decision and relationship in our future. So, if your childhood experience has provided you with the underlying belief that you do not deserve a lot in life, then your ability to manifest what you desire may be held back.

Laying the foundations for the experiences you desire is critical if you want them to last. You've no doubt heard about the high proportion of lottery winners that blow it all in a short period of time; neuroscience would suggest they were not sufficiently primed for the experience. Neuroscientist and author Dr. Joe Dispenza explains:

"The average person has 60,000 to 70,000 thoughts in one day. Out of those 60,000 to 70,000 thoughts that you think in one day, 90 percent of those are the same thoughts as the day before. So, the same thoughts will always lead to the same choices. The same choices will always lead to the same behaviors. The same behaviors will always create the same experiences. And the same experiences always produce the same emotions. Those same emotions drive our very same thoughts and our biology."

Dispenza estimates that 95 percent of who you are by the time you're 35 years old is a memorized state of being. There's a saying in neuroscience that neurons that fire together wire together, in other words, you are what you repeatedly do. The hardest part about creating desirable change is not creating the same thoughts or making the same choices you habitually made the day before.

What I like about Dispenza's work is that he backs up what was once thought to be mystical, with hard science. His team uses MRI, brain scans, Heart Rate Variability testing, as well as testing gene expression, immune regulation, cellular metabolism, and longevity measurements to quantify the processes described here.

Change, even positive change, can feel uncomfortable and unfamiliar. It's hard work to push through those wired-in beliefs and there are neurobiological reasons for that. For most people it takes a tragedy like a major illness or crisis to provide sufficient motivation to create such change. Why wait for a crisis? Wouldn't it be better to create the life you want when you're most physically and psychologically able to enjoy it? By understanding and harnessing some basic principles of neuroscience, particularly those relating to neuroplasticity (the ability for the brain to change) we're able to influence our brains to work for us rather than hold us back.

To create the change you want to see, it's important to become conscious of your unconscious habits and behaviors. The practice of meditation is a powerful tool for creating such self-awareness. Dr. Dispenza explains it something like this: the neural pathways in your brain are laid down in response to events—what you're told, what you see, and what you experience. You can liken it to cutting a path through the jungle to get to a water source. Once you've established that path you continue to use it because it's the easiest way to get to the water and so the path becomes worn from the daily trek. So it is with the brain as it lays its neural networks.

Those neural pathways—our deep-down beliefs about ourselves—can be very hard to shift because that path is well laid and familiar, even if it is awful. Some people wonder how women can stay in abusive relationships or move from one abuser to the next. It might seem unfathomable for those of us who do not have that well-established neural pathway that tells us (subconsciously) that we are not worthy of better treatment.

There are several ways we can deal with our deeply held beliefs and break the cycle of those that don't serve us well. Joe Dispenza speaks about it in terms of pruning synaptic connections and sprouting new ones, un-memorizing emotional states that have become part of your personality and reconditioning your body to a new emotion or to a new mind.

Neuroplasticity allows us to learn new things, train the brain, mentally rehearse new ways of being, embed new thinking through focus and repetition, and reprogram unconscious thoughts. From a purely biochemical view, your brain via the RAS seeks out the experiences and opportunities you desire. It's also known as manifesting. Here's one way you might go about it:

1. Think of a goal

2. Consider it in every aspect and leave nothing out. If you want to make more money, make sure you request it to happen in the best way possible for all concerned. Most importantly, consider how it would make you feel

3. Visualize that goal and see it happening without any impediments

4. Create a mood board with all the elements of the goal and look at it every day and try to feel what would be like to actually have

achieved that goal. This is a crucial point that is often missed. In feeling as if you're already there, you're establishing the neural networks associated with that wanted experience

5. Sit back and watch as your RAS works with your subconscious and conscious mind to make it happen

Maintaining cognitive health is vital because your mind governs the rest of you and the way you think determines everything—the way you relate to others, how well you take care of yourself and others, and the sense of a life well-lived.

If you have been resistant to attending to your poor hearing, it's worth asking yourself why and seeing where that takes you. It might be that you think it means surrendering to ageing, that you will be seen as old, or that you will have to wear some awful, clunky-looking devices in your ears. Then it's worth asking yourself whether these thoughts reflect what is true and whether you can just be realistic about your health and accept the reality rather than be in conflict with it. You might also consider that dealing with your hearing issue will help protect you from cognitive decline, and be reassured by the fact that there is good evidence to suggest that much of such damage can be reversable.

"A man practices the art of adventure when he breaks the chain of routine and renews his life through reading new books, traveling to new places, making new friends, taking up new hobbies."

~Wilfred Arlen Peterson

PART 2

Caring For Cognition

CHAPTER 6

The 1% rule and the aggregate of marginal gains

Luckily, when it comes to solving your hearing issues, it happens with immediate effect, albeit with a period of acclimatization. Once you attach those teeny devices to your ears, you can hear better immediately. Other kinds of life changes, including cognitive repair, take more time to manifest results. Part 2 outlines additional, specific interventions that may be considered supplementary to the advice set out in Part 1. It may help to think of these as 1% tactics that can combine and complement each other over time.

Too often we set a lofty goal only to be disappointed when we fall short, so I like the '1% rule' because it makes everything feel more manageable. By breaking things down into incremental achievements, you can yield remarkable results.

In James Clear's book, *Atomic Habits*, he tells the story of the British cycling team. They hadn't won an Olympic gold medal for 95 years, and no British cyclist had won the Tour De France in 110 years. In fact, one of the main bicycle manufacturers in Europe refused to sell bikes to them in order to preserve their reputation.

Things changed in 2003 when cycling consultant Dave Brailsford was appointed their performance director. Brailsford's strategy centered around the 'aggregate of marginal gains', that is, the concept of searching for small gains in everything you do.

"The whole principle came from the idea that if you broke down everything you could think of that goes into riding a bike, and then improve it by one percent, you will get a significant increase when you put them all together," said Brailsford.

Brailsford and his team set about making one percent gains in a wide range of areas; in both expected and unexpected ways. Expected improvements related to the gear they wore, better gripping tires and the use of biofeedback sensors to track performance. Some of the unconventional improvements included optimization of massage gels, pillow optimization for better sleeping, handwashing training to reduce the risk of catching a cold, and painting the inside of the team truck white to better identify dust that could interfere with finely-tuned bicycles. After making hundreds of adjustments, the results were rapidly enhanced.

- In the 2008 Olympics in Beijing, the British cycling team won an incredible 60% of the gold medals

- In the 2012 Olympics in London, the team set nine Olympic records and seven world records

- Between 2012 and 2018, the Tour de France was won by members of the team five out of six times

The suggestions in this book are only expected to yield results when applied consistently and gradually over the long term. In his book, *The 1% Rule*, Tommy Baker explains the power of this principal. "If you can just consistently and persistently be 1% better at what you do each day, over the course of a year or a decade you will make significant progress."

There are two ways in which this concept may assist us in our efforts towards better cognitive health. Firstly, if we engage in a broad range of interventions, there's a great chance they will complement each other and act as a holistic intervention that is far greater than the sum of its parts. This strategy can be referred to as the aggregate of marginal gains. Secondly, aiming to do just one percent better each day for the things you want to improve, can result in significant progress over time.

"As a single footstep will not make a path on the earth, so a single thought will not make a pathway in the mind. To make a deep physical path, we walk again and again. To make a deep mental path, we must think over and over the kind of thoughts we wish to dominate our lives."

~Wilfred Arlan Peterson

CHAPTER 7

Food for life

We know that most chronic diseases are preventable—heart disease, diabetes, cancer, arthritis, etcetera. Most often they're caused by lifestyle choices: smoking, over-indulgence in alcohol, unmanaged stress.

Preventative medicine is the best medicine, and we all need to take responsibility for doing our best to maintain physical, spiritual, mental, and emotional balance. This can't always be a solitary ondeavor, which is why we engage with health service providers to guide us to make changes. The part we need to play is to become aware of what our body is telling us, and not ignore the slight aches and pains or deficiencies.

Discomfort is our body's way of letting us know when things are out of whack; however, if we don't pay attention, things may get worse. This is especially true when it comes to hearing and brain health.

It's easy to attend a doctor and ask them to fix you, especially when we are very sick or in chronic pain, and need some very quick fixing. If you take another view and make a different commitment to yourself, you might avoid the need for acute or chronic care.

Good nutrition is a given, and there are many ways to eat well. It seems dietary issues and restrictions are perpetually on the rise. New fad diets hit the shelves regularly, all of which are somewhat removed from my audiology wheelhouse. Much has been written on the topic of nutrition and brain health and I'd encourage the interested reader to take a look at *Lifespan* by Dr. David Sinclair, and *End of Alzheimer's* by Dr. Dale Bredesen as a great start.

For now, though, I'll take you on a brief journey into what I've researched as my three top mood and brain-enhancing foods, which could also be described as preventative supplements.

HOT CHOCOLATE: CEREMONIAL CACAO

Core Benefits: Neuroprotective and mood enhancing

"Cacao has the highest antioxidant concentration of any major food in the world. Cacao is thirty times higher in antioxidants than red wine, twenty times more potent in antioxidants than blueberries, three times higher than acai, and twice as much as chaga mushrooms. These antioxidants protect our cells from free radical damage and therefore contribute to our longevity and state of wellbeing."

~David Wolfe

The idea that chocolate is medicine could be music to many ears. Chocolate is made from cacao, which are the seeds that grow inside pods. In their raw state they taste bitter, nothing like a scrummy mint Lindt. A long process involving fermenting, grinding, and heating takes place to form it into cocoa, then it's further processed to create the milk chocolate available on supermarket shelves. By the time it gets to that stage it contains very little of its original health-bestowing goodness.

Cacao is the unrefined cousin of cocoa and consuming it provides quite an array of health benefits. The concentration of antioxidants in cacao is also effective in protecting against oxidative stress, which is understood to be the primary basis of age-related hearing loss. Processing cacao into cocoa causes the loss of between 60-90 percent of its vital, health-bestowing antioxidants.

Antioxidants are important compounds that help defend cells from damage caused by free radicals, which are unstable atoms that cause a myriad of illnesses, as well as symptoms of ageing (including memory loss) and cell damage. They react easily with other molecules and can cause large chain chemical reactions called oxidation leading to oxidative stress, which can increase the risk of chronic diseases such as cancer, heart disease, and Type 2 diabetes.

Cacao has a long history and its healing properties have been documented over the centuries. Since at least the 1400s, cacao was a sacred plant to Mayans and Aztecs. Aztec mythology says that God created man from maize and cacao, among other plants. (Perhaps it's not such an unusual concept; we're all made up of carbon after all.) It's also reported that cacao was used in ritual sacrifices to lift the spirits of those headed for the chop.

You might question the Mayan belief that a hot chocolate would comfort someone who's about to have their head or heart removed, but it does contain some pretty heady substances that can lift the spirits significantly if taken in the right dose.

Following are three compelling cacao studies:

- A study published in *Frontiers in Nutrition* journal analyzed dozens of cacao-flavanol studies on cognition. The team concluded that the evidence to date shows that they help boost general cognition, attention, processing speed and memory.

- A double-blind study of cacao, cognition and aging found that 90 subjects with mild cognitive impairment had significantly better cognitive function including verbal test scores after consuming cacao flavanols for eight weeks.

- In France, a study followed 1,367 subjects over 65 years old for five years to determine if antioxidant flavonoid intake (concentrated in cacao) influenced neuroprotection (a substance that prevents the death of neurons). It concluded that the intake of antioxidant flavonoids is inversely related to the risk of dementia. In other words, it helps prevent it.

Blissful chemistry

Cacao contains happiness-making substances that we can safely enjoy.

- *Serotonin* is a neurotransmitter commonly known as the 'feel-good chemical'. Cacao not only supplies the body with serotonin, it aids the body in producing its own serotonin naturally. Serotonin combats stress and improves our mood by promoting the feelings of comfort, contentment, happiness, relaxation, and wellbeing. It's also delivered in antidepressant medication; selective serotonin reuptake inhibitors (SSRIs) are a commonly prescribed antidepressant to ease symptoms of moderate to severe depression.

- *Phenylethylamine (PEA)* is also known as the 'love chemical' for its association with the giddy excitement one feels when falling in love. When ingested, PEA stimulates the central nervous system to release the body's endorphins. PEA signals the body to promote the sensation of alertness, focus, and mental acuity while elevating one's mood, speeding up metabolism and boosting memory.

- *Anandamide* (from the Sanskrit word Ananda, meaning bliss) is the 'bliss chemical'. It's a neurotransmitter that to date has only been found in cacao and the human brain. Anandamide doesn't put you in a mind-altered state, but it can produce a feeling of euphoria.

In addition to the hearing and brain health benefits, the flavanols in cacao or dark chocolate are useful to nurture the health of your heart. Studies suggest they can lower blood pressure, reduce blood stickiness, improve the responsiveness of blood vessels, and reduce cholesterol.

More chocolatey good news about cacao's constituents

Cacao contains:

- *Theobromine* is an alkaloid chemical that acts as a vasodilator, meaning it relaxes smooth muscle. Benefits of this chemical include enhanced blood flow and oxygenation to the brain in addition to long-term antioxidant properties.

- *Magnesium.* Cacao is also one of the highest plant-based sources of magnesium, which is one of the minerals we are most deficient of in the First World because we don't eat enough green leafy vegetables. The problem is that every cell in the body contains this mineral and requires it to function. Among a whole host of other benefits, magnesium helps increase energy, calms the nerves, aids in digestion, and relieves muscle aches and pains.

- *Calcium.* Cacao has more calcium than cow's milk would you believe? 160mg per 100g vs only 125mg per 100ml of milk.

The best stuff to ingest is raw, minimally processed, organic ceremonial grade Peruvian cacao because it retains the beneficial properties of this amazing plant. Ceremonial cacao contains 40 times the amount of antioxidant flavonoids contained in blueberries—the highest in any plant.

"After water, cacao is the single healthiest substance you can put in your mouth. Plus, it produces the same chemistry in the brain that occurs when we fall in love."

~**Chris Kilham,** *The Medicine Hunter*

Cacao recipe

To prepare your cacao, take 1 cup of hot water, add 1-2 tablespoons of cacao (remember it's potent so go easy on the amount and see how it affects you), sweeten with honey, coconut sugar, maple syrup or panela (optional). Add a dash of cayenne pepper and/or vanilla extract if possible.

Blend all ingredients in a blender that's safe for hot liquids to create a smooth, frothy drink.

Obviously, ceremonial cacao is no longer used in ritual sacrifices to appease the gods. In these more enlightened times people use it in group ceremonies to connect open-heartedly with others, or to gain clarity, for healing purposes and to set intentions for a fulfilled and happy life. It's also a great meditation aid because of its relaxing qualities. If you want to take the experience up a notch, you can try a ceremonial dose, which is around four tablespoons. This may be a little much if you are sensitive to stimulants like caffeine, though pure cacao contains very little caffeine.

One source of high-grade ceremonial cacao that I like is obtained at flykakao.com. It's grown on the lush tropical island of Kauai, Hawaii. It's a little pricey but it's worth it to obtain such a high-quality product.

BLUEBERRIES

Core Benefit: Neuroprotective

"I may never be happy, but tonight I am content. Nothing more than an empty house, the warm hazy weariness from a day spent setting strawberry runners in the sun, a glass of cool sweet milk, and a shallow dish of blueberries bathed in cream. When one is so

tired at the end of a day one must sleep, and at the next dawn there are more strawberry runners to set, and so one goes on living, near the earth. At times like this I'd call myself a fool to ask for more."

~Sylvia Plath

A pack of blueberries a day could keep the gerontologist away. Researchers at examine.com regard them as the only core supplement for memory and focus. (Examine.com is the largest database of nutrition and supplement research on the internet. It analyzes the full body of evidence available to help people make healthy choices.) They state:

"The antioxidant and anthocyanin content of blueberries makes them particularly effective at reducing cognitive decline, supporting cardiovascular health, protecting the liver, and reducing liver fat build up."

Evidence suggest that not only do blueberries improve cognition in people who are experiencing cognitive decline, they can improve cognition in healthy young people.

Their bioactive compounds anthocyanins and pterostilbene have antioxidant properties that can protect the brain and influence its activity. The anthocyanins in blueberries are believed to contribute to the increased activity of neuronal growth factor (NGF), a neuropeptide that helps neurons grow, branch toward each other, and communicate better.

Delicious blueberries are safe and readily available and don't interact negatively with pharmaceuticals.

How to get the best out of blueberries

Studies show three effective ways to consume blueberries for optimal benefits, even if the fresh fruit is out of season or unavailable.

- *Blueberry anthocyanins:* You can buy this as a super-strength blueberry concentrate in capsule form. The recommended dosage is 500–1,000 mg/day, or 1-2 capsules per day. It's available from health food stores or you can obtain it online from health product retailers.

- *Blueberry powder:* Simply stir this into a glass of water, blend it into a smoothie, sprinkle it over your breakfast muesli, or add it to cakes. Recommended dosage is 5.5–11g/day, which provides between 38.5–77mg of anthocyanins. It's available in 100 percent pure powder from health food stores and online health product retailers. Check the ingredients and avoid the ones that are pumped up with other ingredients and fillers.

- Of course, fresh is best. The most delicious way to consume blueberries is to simply pop fresh ones in your mouth. Take 60–120g/day. Add to fruit salad, blend them into a smoothie or simply snack.

LIONS MANE MUSHROOM

Core Benefit: Cognitive enhancement

Who would have thought that a white, eerie looking, globe-shaped fungi with a long shaggy coat of spines could help you remember the word geranium? A symptom of ageing that many middle-aged to older-aged people report is losing even the most common of words. Mild cognitive impairment is also associated with hearing loss. Lion's mane mushrooms (*Hericium erinaceus*) have been widely used in Asia for both culinary and medicinal purposes and research suggests they may offer a range of health benefits, including reduced inflammation and improved cognitive and heart health.

The brain's ability to grow and form new connections typically declines with age, which may explain why mental functioning deteriorates in many older adults. Studies have found that lion's mane mushrooms contain two special compounds that may stimulate the growth of brain cells—hericenones and erinacines.

According to examine.com, animal studies have found that lion's mane may also help protect against Alzheimer's disease. In fact, lion's mane mushroom and its extracts have been shown to reduce symptoms of memory loss in mice, as well as prevent neuronal damage caused by the amyloid-beta plaques that accumulate in the brain during Alzheimer's disease which disrupt normal function.

The ability of lion's mane mushroom to promote nerve growth and protect the brain from Alzheimer's-related damage may explain some of its beneficial effects on brain health. However, it's important to note that most of the research has been conducted on animals or in test tubes. Therefore, more human studies are needed.

While no studies have analyzed whether lion's mane mushroom is beneficial for Alzheimer's disease in humans, it appears to boost mental functioning. A study in older adults with mild cognitive impairment found that consuming three grams of powdered lion's mane mushroom daily for four months significantly improved mental functioning, but these benefits disappeared when supplementation stopped.

My fascination with lion's mane began when I watched an interview with biohacker and lifestyle guru Dave Asprey who outlined the benefits of the mushroom on REM or rapid eye movement (the dream state) sleep. REM sleep is believed to benefit learning, memory, and mood. A lack of REM sleep may have adverse implications for physical and emotional health. Dr. Bredesen indicated that after taking lion's mane, his REM sleep increased from an average of 30 minutes to 90 minutes per night, which is considered ideal for someone sleeping 7-8 hours per night.

I take it in my coffee in the morning and I've achieved a regular 90 minutes of REM sleep per night and better clarity throughout the day (I measure my sleep cycle on my Fitbit). Health food stores sell lion's mane extract in supplement form. I use the same supplement Dave Asprey recommends, which is Lions Mane Liquid Extract made in Byron Bay by Lifecykel.

Please don't consider my nutritional research as a substitute for the professional advice of your doctor, medical specialist, or nutritionist. If in doubt, please consult your doctor. Seek the advice of your health practitioner before modifying your diet or taking natural medicines.

CHAPTER 8

Brain enhancing activities

SLEEP

Core Benefits: Sleeping your way to overall good health

Sleeping isn't an optional activity, it's a vital function that's as important to our health and wellbeing as good nutrition and exercise. Most mammals, birds, reptiles and bugs do it. Rats deprived of sleep seemingly die faster than those deprived of food.

Once we slip into an unconscious state, our body sets about executing a range of vital restorative tasks. Throughout the night, the brain goes through five sleep-cycle stages and if we miss out on any of them, it can have a significant impact on cognitive function, which means your ability to learn and think clearly.

The term insomnia encompasses a range of sleep disturbances from sleep apnea and snoring, to waking up for a pee during the night. It's any circumstance where you have trouble falling asleep, staying asleep or returning to sleep. Whatever your disrupted sleep entails, it interrupts the cycle and the body's restoration process. Around one in three people have some form of sleep disorder in Australia and the United States, and around one in seven have full-on insomnia.

Effects of poor sleep

Just as there's a strong correlation between hearing and memory, people who have troubled sleep have an increased risk of developing hearing loss. This is largely due to cardiovascular issues that may be caused by lack of sleep. One side-effect of insomnia is poor blood circulation, which of course includes your ears. The tiny hair cells in your ears depend on sufficient blood flow. Interruption to this can contribute to hearing loss. It can also exacerbate the rowdiness of tinnitus, and those increased whizzing, whirring, buzzing noises can in turn disrupt sleep—vicious cycle 101.

Sleep apnea causes people to actually stop breathing throughout the night, which also wakes the sufferer.

Apnea, which affects around 43 percent of people with insomnia, presents all kinds of risks including stroke. Studies show that people with sleep apnea often have larger amounts of plaque in their blood vessels, which may further constrict blood flow to the ear's hair cells and thus damage hearing.

Chronic bad sleep also effects hormone production and metabolism, hence it has a similar effect to the ageing process. This can lead to the development of a range of age-related illnesses including loss of memory, Type 2 diabetes, and high blood pressure. Longer-term, it can contribute to cognitive decline including dementia and Alzheimer's.

Regular sleep interruptions affect the part of the brain that controls memory, language and even our sense of time. Deep sleep also has a profound effect on our mental state. Research shows that the parts of the brain that control emotions, decision making, and social interactions appear to be quiet during the deep sleep stage. This suggests they are using that time to recover from all the hard work they do during wakefulness.

Another important function of deep sleep is restoration and recovery, and there's evidence that a flushing process occurs during this stage that may be protective against Alzheimer's disease. Human Growth Hormone (HGH), which helps maintain, build, and repair healthy tissue in the brain and other organs, is also secreted during deep sleep.

Memory and sleep are also intimately linked. Lack of sleep affects our 'working memory', which is an executive function that allows us to call upon information and hold it in place while we solve something complex. Examples of this are holding a mix of consonants and vowels in your mind and then figuring out the words they might construct, or doing an equation in your head and drawing upon other numbers and combinations to find an answer.

During each of the five stages of sleep, different functions occur that get our thoughts organized, filed and consolidated. General findings of various studies show that poor sleep may impair intellectual performance. The NREM (non-rapid eye movement sleep) and REM (rapid eye movement sleep) are important for memory consolidation—where recent learned experiences are turned into long term memories. The brain organizes the information for easy recall. It's believed that NREM sleep is linked with the formation of your declarative memory, that is the part that holds basic facts, events and statistics, and REM sleep boosts your procedural memory, which involves remembering sequences.

We know what it is to sleep on a problem and wake up in the morning with an answer that's been evading us. That's because sleep may also facilitate more complex forms of insight.

Some studies show that sleep deprived people are at risk of forming false memories. They may have a reduced ability to think flexibly and develop poor emotional judgement. Sleep deprivation can also impact our immunity so we become more susceptible to infections, colds and flu, and mental health issues such as anxiety and depression can be exacerbated.

If you need more of a wake-up call in relation to the dangers inherent in lying awake counting blades of grass, imagine this: being awake for 17 consecutive hours is equivalent to the impairment caused by drinking two glasses of wine.

In summary, a bad night's sleep can seriously diminish your ability to concentrate, communicate effectively, handle complex tasks, think logically, make good decisions and be creative. However, don't panic, the odd night spent tossing and turning will unlikely set you on a downward spiral, although you may have some temporary impairment.

As well as poor sleep making us less than effective thinkers, we are also more likely to make mistakes, which could be fatal. Operating heavy machinery while sleep deprived is a big no-no. Some industries have been hugely impacted by sleep-deprived workers where disastrous, avoidable accidents have occurred. American Airlines Flight 1420 is a case in point. Just before midnight, June 1, 1999, it overshot the runway at Little Rock National Airport killing 10 passengers and the captain with more than a hundred others injured. Investigators found that the pilots probably made the mistake because of tiredness, plus the stress of trying to land the plane during a thunderstorm.

Then there's the *Challenger* shuttle explosion, the *Exxon Valdez* spill, the nuclear disaster at Chernobyl and the melting of the nuclear reactor core at Three Mile Island. All of these have been attributed to sleep deprivation. At a more relatable level, sleeplessness causes around 25 percent of road accidents, loss of productivity in the workplace, and even marriage and relationship breakdowns.

Given the risks involved with developing poor sleep habits, it's a good idea to do something about it before you head steadily and wakefully down the road of emotional, intellectual, and physical decline.

Causes of sleep issues

How high is up and how many causes are there of sleeplessness, are similar types of questions. It's relatively common for people to experience insomnia at one time or another such as during stressful periods or illness. However, eventually, normal sleep patterns return. It becomes serious when a disrupted sleep pattern sets in on a regular basis.

Insomnia can develop due to ill health, electromagnetic radiation, jet lag, physiological, psychological and hormonal problems, stress, or food allergies. Women are more likely candidates than men for a variety of reasons. The elderly and depressed are also more susceptible.

Following are some factors that are likely to keep you awake at night:

• Pharmaceutical medications including anti-hypertensive drugs, weight loss drugs, pseudoephedrine, the oral contraceptive pill, corticosteroids (for inflammatory conditions), Parkinson's disease medications and antidepressants

- Recreational drug use

- Nicotine

- Caffeine is a stimulant. It's in black tea, coffee, cocoa, and soft drinks. Best not to drink coffee from late afternoon

- Alcohol might get you off to sleep, but it also impairs sleep because it decreases the time spent in the REM cycle and causes sleep disturbance in the second half of the sleep period. It's best to avoid alcohol within two to three hours of bedtime. It also causes the release of adrenaline and weakens the transport of tryptophan into the brain. The brain is dependent on tryptophan as the source for serotonin (the neurotransmitter that initiates sleep) and alcohol disrupts serotonin levels

- Poor lifestyle habits such as playing video games or working before going to bed and not taking time to wind down and relax

How to establish and maintain good sleep patterns

If you want to function optimally, think clearly, make good decisions without feeling the need for a nanna nap, you need a regular sleep pattern. You could take sleeping pills and sedatives such as benzodiazepines if you're suffering from chronic insomnia. These may be helpful in the short term but they can be addictive and you can develop a tolerance so you have to rely on higher doses. Further, sleep medications tend to reduce the proportion of restorative deep sleep in most people.

This is an area where technology offers some exciting solutions. Several smartphone app-driven devices are available that can assist in monitoring your sleep cycles, and they also provide advice. This means you can track not only the quantity, but the quality of sleep you're getting.

Some sleep tracking options you may consider are the Apple watch, Fitbit, Whoop Strap or Oura Ring. In addition, the Muse S brain sensing headband is a meditation aid that has a comprehensive sleep tracking function. It tracks brainwave, heart rate, breath, and movement to give deep insights into your sleep quality.

There are also new technologies that help stimulate sleep. NeoRhthym is a neurostimulation headband that uses pulsed electromagnetic field (PEMF) technology to help entrain your desired state of mind. For example, delta brain waves are known to be associated with deep or slow-wave sleep. The NeoRhythm headband has a sleep setting that pulses at delta frequencies to help safely influence this state in the brain. Using this 20 minutes before bedtime in a specific position on the head readies the brain for sleep. You then place it under your pillow for eight hours. This device has increased my deep sleep time by an average of half an hour each night.

There are other settings on the NeoRhythm for focused attention, alertness, relaxation, meditation and even pain control.

Tips for getting a good night's sleep:

• Bedrooms should be for sleep and loving, intimate relations. They're not an office

• Make sure the bedroom is comfortable (warm, but not too hot), pillow and bedding are comfortable, the room is dark

- Lavender oil on the temples (not suitable for children)

- Meditation

- A relaxing bath before bed with some lovely calming essential oils such as lavender, ylang ylang, sandalwood and orange

- There are herbal and homeopathic concoctions in the marketplace, however it's worthwhile getting advice from a qualified health practitioner so you choose something that is right for your body

- Herbal teas such as chamomile, rosemary and passionflower are helpful

- Listen to beautiful sounds online such as the sea or rain

- Avoid watching a violent or scary movie before bed. Part of creating a good atmosphere to sleep involves a calm environment and mindset

- Avoid drinking a lot of water or other beverages before bed

Eating for sleep

Our digestive system slows down at night in favor of the many vital restorative functions the body undertakes while we sleep. A late, heavy meal will therefore be harder to digest and is likely to keep you awake.

The best after-dinner snack is something containing high protein because protein is made from amino acids such as tryptophan, which is the precursor for melatonin and serotonin.

If you do need a late snack, eat food that contains complex carbohydrates and protein to optimize tryptophan levels. A warm glass of milk with a dash of honey could be just the ticket to slumberland. Other foods that aid sleep include walnuts, almonds, turkey, tuna, bananas and kiwifruit. Calcium also helps release serotonin so milk, sesame and sunflower seeds, broccoli, oats and tahini are helpful.

Generally avoid bad quality/refined carbohydrates like white bread and biscuits, which can raise blood-sugar levels and cause a burst of energy that makes us more likely to dance than sleep. Soft drinks, spicy food (think heartburn and indigestion), alcohol, caffeine, monosodium glutamate (MSG is a stimulant), and foods containing additives, preservatives and pesticides, are all to be avoided if you want to sleep well. Regardless of sleep, none of these substances are going to do you any good.

PLAY MUSIC

Core Benefits: Cognitive, mood and motor enhancement

"If music be the food of love, play on."

~William Shakespeare, *Twelfth Night*

The strong relationship between music training and cognitive performance is well established. Studies have shown that people with instrumental music training have enhanced neurological and cognitive processing compared to those who are not engaged in playing.

We know that music lessons are wonderful for children's brains because they can significantly enhance their abilities in relation to verbal ability, language, reasoning, and memory. The same applies to adults.

Playing a musical instrument involves the engagement of multiple components of the brain. Playing an instrument engages the brain's motor systems—the central and peripheral brain structures in the nervous system that are involved in initiating movements. This enables the activation of the gross and fine movements required to produce the sounds. In addition, sensory information from the fingers, hands and arms is sent to the brain for processing.

There are memory and pattern recognition components involved as well. If the musician is reading music, visual information is sent to the brain for processing and interpreting commands for the motor centers. Then there are our emotional responses to the music, which are processed by the brain. Being in a group or band and playing to an audience can have further emotional and social benefits.

If lack of hearing is affecting your memory, then learning to play a musical instrument or joining a choir may be a great activity to strengthen your cognitive abilities.

Music's affect on the brain is well-studied. On

functional MRI scans, the brain lights up like a Christmas tree in response to music.

- Researchers at the University of Southern California investigated 157 pairs of older twins. In controlling for sex, education, and physical activity, playing a musical instrument was significantly associated with less likelihood of dementia and cognitive impairment compared to their co-twin

- A study at the Heriot-Watt University in Edinburgh researched the differences between musicians and non-musicians aged 60–93 years old across a range of neuropsychological measures of cognitive function. Musicians performed significantly better than non-musicians in all domains

Related to both physical exercise and music are the brain health benefits of dance. Several studies have shown that dancing (particularly ballroom dancing and salsa) is linked to a reduced risk of dementia.

- Researchers at the Albert Einstein College of Medicine found that dancing is associated with 76 percent reduced risk of dementia

- A study published in the *Frontiers in Aging Neuroscience* journal shows that dancing improves intellectual health and spatial memory

Aside from the brain benefits, dancing's great fun and it makes dancers feel happy.

My passion for music was one of the core reasons I decided to become an audiologist. I played bass guitar in bands right through high school and during my undergraduate psychology studies. My exposure to various amplified guitar and public address systems gave me insight into acoustic principals, the workings of the inner ear, and the 'ear' to fine tune hearing devices. It's not such a wide stretch between playing amplified music and hearing devices; after all, hearing aids have a microphone, processor, amplifier and speaker, albeit on a smaller scale.

LANGUAGE LEARNING

Core Benefit: Cognitive enhancement

Learning a language is not just a mechanical act, it widens our world view and engages us with new cultures and ideas. It's been shown that people who speak more than one language often exhibit more empathy and a global mindset. Researchers report that some people even feel like a different person while speaking their second language.

Your brain thrives on learning new and complex things. Learning another language is one of the most novel and challenging activities you can do. In my first book, *Hearing & Brain Health*, I described some of the insights from leading neuroscientist Lisa Genova who endorses the deliberate engagement in new experiences to build new connections in our brains. If we consider Alzheimer's, for instance, which can be incubating for 25 years before one becomes symptomatic, that disease acts on existing connections. However, as Lisa Genova explains, consistent novelty and challenge can build fresh connections in the brain effectively building a buffer, a form of resilience against cognitive decline.

She advocates learning a new language, going to new places, meeting new people, and learning new skills. A second language not only has direct cognitive benefits, it may also open up all kinds of novel possibilities with travel and exposure to other cultures.

• Research published in the *American Journal of Neurology*, demonstrated that knowing a second language can postpone the onset of dementia and Alzheimer's by an impressive 4.5 years

• In a study published in medical journal *Annals of Neurology*, researchers found that those who spoke two or more languages had significantly better cognitive abilities compared to what would have been expected from their baseline test. The strongest effects were seen in general intelligence and reading. These effects were present in those who had learned their second language early as well as later in life

• A study titled, 'The Cognitive Benefits of Being Bilingual' published in the *Cerebrum Journal*, showed that the bilingual brain can have better focus and task-switching capacities than the monolingual brain, because it has developed the ability to inhibit one language while using another. This research also found that bilingual seniors can experience less cognitive decline

I've been fortunate to have lived and worked in several countries; as a child in Papua New Guinea, as an audiologist/manager in Singapore, Malaysia and Taiwan, and as a traveler in Europe and South America. It's important to enjoy the language you're learning and there's no substitute for speaking it regularly.

My favorite way of learning another language is via the Pimsleur audiobook language courses because they have you speaking the language straight away. If you have the opportunity to immerse yourself in an environment where you have no choice but to speak the language, that will really fast track your progress.

"The art of conversation lies in listening."

~Malcolm Forbes

BRAIN TRAINING

Core Benefit: Cognitive enhancement

If you understand the principles of neuroplasticity, you'll know that the brain has the potential to grow new connections and rewrite its story. Doctors once believed the brain didn't change after around the age of 17. The opposite was found to be true; the brain is in constant flux. Neuroplasticity is a dynamic set of processes that occur at any age.

Neuroplasticity happens in adults in three ways: by forming new connections whenever you learn something new, strengthening existing connections through repeating an activity, and removing or reducing unused pathways. Keeping the brain from shutting down any functions, especially as we age, may take some effort. If you have the added issue of hearing loss, which affects the part of the brain associated with memory and cognitive function, it's time to break out the brain fitness activities.

A substantial study on longevity out of Pew Research Center in Washington DC indicates that only 20 percent of respondents wanted to live to age 90 or older. They had this attitude largely due to concerns about decline in health and, in particular, dementia.

According to Alexandre Bennett, a clinical neuropsychologist who specializes in geriatrics, the fear of dementia is often greater than the fear of death itself.

"People fear this more than death because it steals your personality and turns you into somebody that requires total care," she says.

We know that undertaking physical exercise at least three times a week is advisable for overall wellbeing, longevity, and prevention of decline. When you build strength in the gym or lose a few kilos, you can see the physical changes in the mirror or by checking back to past photos. Improvements in our cognitive abilities, however, are more or less invisible in the absence of obvious behavioral signs.

The notion of training the mind on a similar regimen may seem odd but there are some terrific, scientifically proven online mind training technologies specifically for enhancing cognitive abilities. They are easy, accessible, and highly motivating.

Before we dive into those, I must point out the impact that treating hearing loss has on cognition. Recent studies published by the University of Maryland and University of Melbourne on specific measures of cognition including short term memory, processing speed, and executive function (the ability of the brain to regulate mental processes that enable us to remember instructions, plan, focus attention, and multitask) showed improvement after six months of full-time quality hearing device use. This adds to the growing body of evidence regarding the effect that hearing devices have on cognitive function.

When training the mind, Sudoku and crossword puzzles can be helpful, however they're limited in scope. A major study in the *British Medical Journal* found that crosswords and Sudoku could boost mental ability in specific ways, but they had no influence over mental decline as people age. The skills that are achieved in these activities are very specific, but eventually plateau and progress is limited. It's like going to the gym and performing a couple of specific exercises with the same weight; you'll reach a point where progress flattens out.

In relation to the association between cognitive training and audiology, consider your ability to hear in background noise. This involves separating the target signal, which are those things you want to hear, from distracting background noise. Then there's an interplay between pattern recognition, which is the cognitive process that matches information from a stimulus such as something someone has said, with information that already lies in your memory. For instance, when you don't hear all the consonants in a word, and you take your recognition cues from what you already know and guess.

The most common forms of hearing loss results in a loss of perception of many higher-pitch consonant sounds. If it's not treated, we compensate with visual input, including body language, facial expression and lip movement (lip reading) to fill in the gaps. This is a considerable and multifaceted cognitive task and so taxing on the brain that it one of the core links between untreated hearing loss and cognitive decline. Brain training can go a long way to helping to address this, providing it's applied consistently.

- A study published in 2018, by the *Journal of the American Geriatrics Society* found that brain training may help people with mild cognitive impairment (MCI), and the stage between normal brain ageing and dementia. They recruited 145 adults diagnosed with MCI (average age 72).

They were split into three groups; one did two hours of brain training focused on improving memory every week for two months. The second did two hours of training per week focused on the positive aspects of their lives, and learning how to cope with stress and frustration. The third group didn't have a program. The people in the brain training group scored two to four times higher on tests and maintained their improvement over a six-month period

• Recent research published by Edith Cowan University examined 26 peer-reviewed studies on the effectiveness of seven brain training programs for people aged over 50. They found two programs that reached the gold standard— Level 1 in scientific backing. These are Cognifit and BrainHQ.

After reviewing close to 8,000 studies, reviewers at the University of Western Australia stated that CogniFit brain training possessed the highest level of evidence of concrete positive effects for healthy ageing. CogniFit is classified as a cognitively preventative program for dementia, i.e., a serious game that keeps the player cognitively engaged and slows the symptoms.

If you engage in Cognifit, I'd encourage you to do it regularly but don't become dependent on that alone for enhancing and protecting your cognitive health. Good evidence shows that taking a multidisciplinary or holistic approach is likely to yield even better results in cognitive tests. For instance, in one study, older people who use CogniFit and combine it with physical activity, improve their cognitive state more than those who only do physical activity or who only read. Another study showed strong links between cognitive, social and physiological areas, which makes a case for a holistic approach to enhancing and assessing wellness.

Cognifit consists of a general cognitive assessment component and provides a personalized training program. The assessment generates an overall score out of 800 and an equivalent cognitive age based on your results. As you progress through the training program, which is simply 15-20 minutes every second day, your score out of 800 changes. I have to say that I find it quite motivating to see my score improve (on most days!). I'd encourage you to give it a try. You have nothing to lose and so much to potentially gain.

If you have serious concerns about your cognitive

health, I'd encourage you to discuss this with your doctor. Alternatively, you can find further information on the following comprehensive website, **www. dementia.org.au.**

TAPPING

Core Benefits: Stress and pain reduction, eases depression and anxiety, lowers cortisol levels, helps clear trauma, releases fears and negative habits

Based on the combined principles of ancient Chinese acupressure and modern psychology, the modality of 'tapping', also known as EFT (Emotional Freedom Techniques), is a powerful holistic healing tool. Increasing evidence from research demonstrates its efficacy in helping to resolve a range of issues including stress, anxiety, phobias, emotional disorders, chronic pain, addiction, weight control, and limiting beliefs, just to name a few. Research shows that tapping can also lower cortisol levels.

It works on the level of stimulating acupoints

(think acupuncture without needles), which sends signals to the amygdala in the limbic system—the part of the brain involved in behavioral, fear and emotional responses. EFT also appears to affect the hippocampus (memory center), particularly in its interaction with the amygdala.

Literally tapping parts of your body with two fingertips on specific meridian points (pressure points) on the face and upper body, while focusing on particular negative emotions or physical sensations, helps to calm the nervous system and influence or 'rewire' the brain to respond in healthier ways.

There are eight tapping points:

1. Start of the eyebrow (in the middle of the brows)

2. Side of the eye

3. Under the eye

4. Under the nose

5. Directly under the lips

6. 2.5cm under the collarbone

7. Under the arm in line with the nipple

8. Centre of the head.

At the same time as gently tapping each of those points in turn, you repeat a phrase that sums up how you're feeling, such as 'I feel hurt, I feel hurt' or 'I feel angry, I feel angry'. This might seem odd but by repeatedly expressing how you feel while tapping for around 5-10 minutes, you will feel the emotion or stress ease because it changes the cortisol levels.

- At Bond University a study led by clinical and health psychologist, Associate Professor Peta Stapleton, compared the effects on cortisol levels of an hour of tapping compared with spending that time reading magazines or being taught about stress and how it impacts the body. The tapping group had a 43 percent reduction in cortisol compared with a 19.5 percent drop in cortisol in those who learned about stress, and a two percent reduction for those who read magazines

EFT has also been researched at a physiological level, including its effects on genes. An initial pilot study using four participants compared an hour-long EFT session with a placebo session, where subjects thought they were getting a treatment; however, it didn't have an active component. This small study revealed incredible information. After the single EFT session there was differential expression in 72 genes associated with:

• The suppression of cancer tumors

• Protection against ultraviolet radiation

• Regulation of Type 2 diabetes insulin resistance

• Immunity from opportunistic infections

• Antiviral activity

• Synaptic connectivity between neurons

• Synthesis of both red and white blood cells

• Enhancement of male fertility

• Building white matter in the brain

• Metabolic regulation

• Neural plasticity

• Reinforcement of cell membranes

• Reduction of oxidative stress

Since then, another study involving 16 war veterans with PTSD who received 10 hour-long EFT sessions, examined how this affected the regulation of six genes associated with inflammation and immunity.

After EFT treatment, interleukins, which are responsible for regulating our body's inflammation response, decreased significantly in expression. The 'good' genes associated with improved functioning of the immune system were up-regulated (expressed). There was also a significant association between improvement in the veterans' mental-health symptoms and positive changes in the expression of their genes related to stress hormones.

There are no reported side effects from tapping, and a formal research study of 1,000 people who experienced trauma demonstrated there were no reported adverse reactions to using EFT.

EFT has been particularly effective in relation to tinnitus. A good EFT practitioner can work with you to determine the underlying issue that precipitated the onset of the tinnitus, and then the tapping can help release those emotion blockages at the source.

Whilst tapping is self-administered, if you want to further investigate this very useful modality, it's a good idea to consult a qualified practitioner who can guide you through the process and help you understand the related emotional issues.

Associate Professor Peta Stapleton has written a comprehensive book on the subject called *The Science of Tapping*, outlining in greater detail the technique and the scientific studies supporting its effectiveness.

BEING IN NATURE AND GROUNDING

Core Benefits: Anti-inflammatory, stress reduction and sleep quality

More than a thousand studies have been conducted on the importance of being in nature for physical, emotional, and cognitive wellbeing. It can lower blood pressure and stress hormone levels, calm your nervous system, enhance the function of your immune system, reduce anxiety, and all-round improve your disposition.

It might surprise you to know that gardening can improve your mental health. A meta-analysis of research published in the journal *Preventative Medicine Reports*, found that it can reduce depression and anxiety. Digging in the dirt stirs up microbes in the soil that when inhaled stimulate serotonin production, which makes you feel relaxed and content. Digging the spuds and carrots creates psychological and physical wellbeing, and even improves cognitive function.

- Researchers at the European Centre for Environment and Human Health at the University of Exeter studied almost 20,000 people across various occupations, income brackets and ethnicities, including those with disabilities and chronic illnesses. They found that those who spent two hours a week in nature, whether it be in parks, at the beach, or in the bush, were substantially more likely to report good health and psychological wellbeing than those who don't

- A study out of the University of Michigan showed that people who walked in nature performed 20 percent better on a memory test than those who walked in the city.

So, it's official, being in nature is good for you!

Grounding

One reason being in nature is so good for you is because it's grounding; you're physically connected with the Earth. Grounding (sometimes known as earthing) is a therapeutic technique that requires no skill other than the ability to remove your shoes and socks. It involves having direct contact with the Earth for 30-40 minutes per day or the use of a grounding device, like my super nerdy grounded pillowcase, which I've found has improved my sleep immeasurably.

The ancient Egyptians, Indigenous Australians, and Native Americans believed in the healing power of interacting directly with the Earth It's believed that the gentle electrical energy the earth emits stabilizes our bioelectrical systems.

Subtle, negative electrical charges exist in the Earth's surface due to lightning strikes and atmospheric pressure. Atomically speaking, the earth is full of free electrons, which are the smallest unit of negative charge. This negative charge can positively affect the normal functioning of all body systems such as the heartbeat and nervous systems, which rely on electrical impulses, and the biological clock, circadian rhythms and cortisol levels.

The phenomenon has been studied for more than 20 years with results published in several peer reviewed journals. By connecting our bare feet with the Earth, we are communing with those charges and helping our bodies in a myriad of ways including improving sleep and reducing pain. Stress levels are impacted through regulating cortisol—it shifts the body from the stressed fight or flight mode to the restorative rest-and-digest mode. Blood circulation is enhanced, as is the immune system, inflammation is decreased, and free radicals are neutralized.

Just think back to your last beach holiday. You probably slept better after being barefoot on the beach. Chances are your bare feet hadn't been in touch with the Earth for some time.

For more information on grounding, there are free books and documentaries available at grounded.com and ultimatelongevity.com, as well as links to over 20 peer reviewed scientific studies.

ESSENTIAL OILS

Core benefits: Reduction of stress and anxiety, adjunctive aid in some health conditions, cognitive enhancement

It's been documented as far back as the 12th century that flowers have been distilled for healing purposes in both Persia and Spain. These days, essential oils, so called because they distil the essence of the plant's fragrance, are used largely for their relaxing qualities. However, they've also been found to be useful for enhancing cognition and dealing with anxiety.

Essential oils can have a positive effect on the mind and body. Preliminary studies demonstrate that essential oils can assist memory and focus; however, scientific research has not yet fully understood the mechanisms. Given that many of our pharmaceutical medicines are taken from nature, this is not such a far stretch.

- A recent study undertaken by scientists from the UK and Duke University set out to determine the effects of essential oils on cognitive performance. They analyzed the ability of numerous essential oils to bind to key receptors and enzymes in the brain that modulate cognitive performance. Preliminary testing identified spearmint and peppermint oils as the most promising because they could bind to two neurotransmitters

- Then they did a double-blind, placebo-controlled, cross-over clinical trial on 24 healthy people. Some were given placebo capsules, others were distributed capsules containing 1 or 2 drops of peppermint or spearmint essential oils. Participants were asked to perform tasks that tested cognitive function, and were assessed for mental fatigue. They discovered that peppermint essential oil had a positive effect on cognition while carrying out challenging mental tasks, and that it significantly reduced cognitive fatigue

Be aware that anything in nature that is therapeutic has the potential to interact adversely with pharmaceutical drugs, so consult with your healthcare provider before using them, and remember that they are generally not to be ingested, only used in a diffuser or on the skin at pulse points.

As a gift to patients, I sometimes provide a long-burn, custom-made candle that my team, an experienced candlemaker and I helped research and develop. We offer either a 'Relationship Harmony' or 'Cognitive Wellness' candle, both of which are infused with a unique blend of essential oils that reinforce our focus on connection and cognition.

The Relationship Harmony candle is a beautiful combination of rose, patchouli, ylang ylang and amber oils, all of which can help with cognitive health and mood. Ylang ylang can help ease the symptoms of anxiety and depression, and as a therapeutic oil, it can assist with releasing trauma and allowing emotional healing so that joy can be felt once more. One study demonstrated that inhalation of ylang ylang had a calming effect because it reduced systolic and diastolic blood pressure significantly. It can also decrease your heart rate, which is helpful if you're anxious with heart pounding. Ylang ylang also has a compound called linalool, which has antibacterial, antifungal, and anti-inflammatory properties.

It takes around 242,000 hand-picked rose petals to produce just 5mL of rose essence. Roses, being the symbol of love, are known for helping to heal the heart and for boosting the immune system. The Persians distilled rosewater into essential oil during the Middle Ages, and rose extracts were renowned throughout Europe, Asia, and the Middle East for improving the complexion.

A 2015 study of postoperative children who inhaled either almond oil or rose oil found that the group who inhaled rose oil reported a significant decrease in their pain levels. Researchers think the rose oil may have stimulated the brain to release endorphins and suggest that aromatherapy using rose oil could be an effective way to ease pain in post-surgery patients.

The musky, earthy fragrance of patchouli aids relaxation, eases stress, depression and anxiety and has been used to treat skin conditions such as acne, dermatitis, and dry skin. It can also aid stomach upsets, colds and headaches among other issues, but it should never be ingested.

Our Cognitive Wellness candle is a blend of lemongrass, cypress, fir needle and leafy green tea. Cyprus oil has a centuries long reputation of being an antiseptic, it's also known to be helpful in pain relief. There's not a large body of research behind this oil, however what has been done is positive.

- In 2007, researchers in Egypt isolated the compounds in cypress leaves and tested them on rat livers. They discovered the antioxidant action protected the rats' livers, so cypress essential oil may be useful to support the liver and as a general antioxidant

- Research undertaken in 2015 showed that cypress oil is high in flavonoids, including a potent antioxidant called quercetin. It can also act as a BChE inhibitor, which prevents the breakdown of a critical neurotransmitter in the brain. This is used in Alzheimer's drugs and indicates that cypress oil may helpful in preventing neurological diseases.

Fir essential oil is extracted through a process of steam distillation from fir needles, which contain the majority of active chemicals and compounds. The earthy scent is known for helping with coughs, colds and respiratory infections and pain. It also has antibacterial and antimicrobial properties.

- A study of fir needles antibacterial activity was published in *Phytotherapy Research* journal, which established that when used to combat Escherichia coli and Staphylococcus aureus, the fir needle essential oil contained three constituents that actively fought the infections

Native Americans used fir needles to pad their pillows to aid peaceful sleep. When fir needle essential oil is diffused or inhaled, it is said to have a grounding and empowering effect that stimulates the mind while relaxing the body.

Green tea is renowned for its antioxidant qualities and as an aid to digestion. Green tea essential oil is great for detoxifying and has many applications including antibacterial, antiviral, and antiseptic qualities. Green tea has been used in traditional Chinese and Indian medicines for such issues as controlling bleeding, wound healing, digestion and heart and mental health. It's thought to aid weight loss, skin conditions, cancer (countries where green tea is consumed regularly have lower cancer rates), and conditions such as liver disorders, Type 2 diabetes and Alzheimer's disease.

- In 2011, researchers conducted a test tube study of the effect of a component of green tea called colon-available green tea extract (CAGTE) to see how it affected a key protein in Alzheimer's disease. Researchers discovered that when it was delivered at high concentration levels, CAGTE protected the cells from the damaging free radicals and beta-amyloid peptides that may play a role in the development of Alzheimer's disease

Not only do these candles have great properties, but they smell divine. If you're interested, you can find out more about them on our NeuAudio website.

"Living is about capturing the essence of things. I go through my life every day with a vial, a vial wherein can be found precious essential oils of every kind. The priceless, fragrant oils are the essence of my experiences, my thoughts...."

~C. JoyBell C.

CHAPTER 9

Keeping fit

Core Benefits: Anti-inflammatory, mood enhancing, stress reduction, cognitive enhancement and social benefits

*"Take care of your body.
It's the only place you have to live in."*

~Jim Rohn

Factors such as poor diet or the modern sedentary lifestyle are detrimental to our health, but they're easy enough to address. If you've ever been lost in the fog of domestic activities or work demands, and taken a brisk walk or a yoga class you'll know how good you feel at the end of it, and how you can return to your duties with a renewed sense of energy and optimism. Exercising, dancing, playing golf or doing yoga creates chemical changes in the brain. Regular, sensible, and appropriate exercise improves blood flow, thinking skills and memory, and reduces the risk of having a stroke or developing heart disease and diabetes.

Exercise can reduce fatigue, improve concentration, and even act like an antidepressant. The runner's high is a well-known effect whereby euphoric feelings result from sustained exercise. In this circumstance, anxiety is reduced and there's a drop in stress hormones.

Several studies have demonstrated the effects of exercise on different parts of the brain. Research by the Department of Exercise Science at the University of Georgia revealed that exercising for 20 minutes aids memory and information processing. Working-out increases our heart rate so more oxygen is pumped to the brain. A variety of hormones are also released during exercise that facilitate the growth of brain cells and stimulate the growth of new connections between cells in a wide array of important cortical areas, thereby enhancing neuroplasticity.

Researchers at Harvard University have also established that exercise helps memory and thinking. Exercise can reduce insulin resistance and inflammation and stimulate the release of growth factors, which are chemicals in the brain that affect the health of brain cells. A run around the block, or a brisk meander around the park will aid the growth of new blood vessels in the brain and help maintain both the abundance and survival of new brain cells.

Exercise helps reduce stress and anxiety and improves mood and sleep. As we know, lack of sleep and mood disorders such as depression frequently cause or contribute to cognitive impairment.

Many studies suggest that the parts of the brain that control thinking and memory are larger in volume in people who exercise than in those who don't. Researchers at the University of British Columbia found that regular aerobic exercise appears to increase the size of the hippocampus, the area of your brain associated with forming new memories and learning. Conversely, resistance training, balance and muscle toning exercises didn't have the same effect.

Other studies suggest that the parts of the brain that control thinking and memory (the prefrontal cortex and medial temporal cortex) are of a greater volume in people who exercise versus people who don't.

Dr. Scott McGinnis, a neurologist at Brigham and

Women's Hospital and an instructor in neurology at Harvard Medical School, was reported on the Harvard Health Publishing site as saying, "...engaging in a program of regular exercise of moderate intensity over six months or a year is associated with an increase in the volume of selected brain regions."

An exercise activity that's effective for people from childhood to senior years is rebounding. It's an activity carried out on a small trampoline or 'rebounder' and it's proven to be a boon for your brain and general health.

Rebounding is a cellular workout, which means it's the only exercise that works every cell in the body as well as your internal organs because it activates your lymphatic system and detoxes the body. While bouncing you are opposing gravity on a vertical plane—the harder the downward bounce the greater the gravitational force. The anti-gravity action of bouncing on a trampoline circulates oxygen to all the tissues and strengthens the nerve pathways between the right and left brain.

Bouncing also increases lymphatic flow as much as fourteen times normal, which helps create a stronger immune system and detoxifies your body.

It can also improve arthritis, osteoporosis (exercise builds bone strength), vision, circulation, balance and coordination. It can also reduce headaches, cholesterol, obesity, slow the ageing process, reduce the risk of cardiovascular disease, and help with sleep.

You absorb more oxygen through exercising, which is helpful in the case of Alzheimer's, dementia, heart disease, diabetes, obesity, and high blood pressure. In addition, exercise stimulates nerve cells to produce chemicals (neurotrophic factors) that stimulate new brain cell growth. These chemicals encourage the brain cells to connect with other neurons.

Sweating, too, is detoxifying and can have beneficial effects on brain health. Dr. Dale Bredesen advocates regular visits to the sauna, whereby research indicates a 66 percent reduced risk of dementia by using a sauna four to seven times per week. Hot yoga is also a great way to keep fit and sweat out those nasty toxins.

Throughout the ageing process our bodies lose muscle mass and bone density. The research tells us that from the age of 30, people can lose up to five percent of muscle mass each decade. It's possible to circumvent that process and remain young until you die of old age, and a growing body of people train to make sure they can maintain good health and vitality throughout their entire lives.

Canadian-American surgeon, Dr. Peter Attia, is one such aspiring centenarian whose medical practice is focused on longevity. He devised activities that would allow him to live the life he wanted when he was a centenarian, and he advises people to decide on what they would still like to be able to do at age 100 and beyond so they can work towards those goals.

These self-styled 'Centenarian Olympics' are a set of personal goals. Your goals might be to maintain the ability to get yourself off the ground if you fall, carry your own shopping into the house, and chase your grandchildren around the yard. The thing is that people tend to expect that growing old means becoming decrepit. I think it's best not to grow and develop that neural pathway. Think about what you would like to achieve in your later years and how you might begin that journey now, no matter your age.

Personally, I like listening to audio books as I take a long walk, or to walk with friends and family. I cycle to work for low impact cardio. My weight training keeps up my strength and bone density, and the feeling afterward is fantastic. I do Yin Yoga for flexibility and relaxation, practice mindfulness meditation and take a sauna when I can. And yes, I have time to work too. Remember, you lose it if you don't use it.

A word of warning: engaging in any activities could be dangerous if you have untreated hearing loss. A nationwide health survey conducted by the Centers for Disease Control and Prevention (USA) showed that hearing impaired people who were tracked for driving, work, and sport and leisure injuries experienced a higher degree of injury risk according to the amount of hearing loss:

- Mild hearing loss – 60% more likely to sustain injury

- Moderate hearing loss – 70% more likely to sustain injury

- Major loss – 90% more likely to sustain injury

Conclusion

A NEW COMMITMENT

With advancements in imaging and research technologies, I anticipate that over the coming years we'll learn more about how we can retain and improve our cognitive health and nurture the marvel between our ears. Given that hearing loss is linked to risk of dementia, let alone the other issues it can cause, and the fact that the simple act of wearing hearing aids 12-16 hours a day can help mitigate those risks, it's exciting to me that we have this power over our wellbeing.

Hearing loss has been identified by peer reviewed scientific journals as the number one modifiable risk factor for the prevention of dementia. Fortunately, hearing loss is highly treatable thanks to today's technology and our increased understanding of how to best manage it.

Then there's the new age of hearing aids, which are now barely discernible, and have joined the world of modern conveniences by linking via Bluetooth to phones and televisions. They're continually evolving, and it seems that in the not-too-distant future their artificial intelligence capability will see them further linked to all kinds of apps and even give us super, substantially better than normal hearing. But for now, they're doing a mighty fine job of restoring hearing and reducing strain on the brain.

I'm proud when I consider the hundreds of lives I've helped change. However, whilst the benefits of treating hearing loss can be profound, it's not the whole story. In effectively dealing with health, body parts should not be considered in isolation. Whilst my wheelhouse remains firmly in the field of audiology, staying abreast of insights that benefit cognitive health is a passion where the benefits flow from me to you.

The whole point of this book is about taking life to another level, not just settling for feeling less than optimum but embracing what you have and living in a state of appreciation of life and its teachings. This is flourishing. It's easy to hang onto our old ways, no matter how difficult they might be because they are familiar and feel safer. Hopefully, this won't be the end of your story. Hopefully, this book will inspire you to take on and explore whatever modalities resonate with you so that you can achieve and maintain optimum physical and cognitive health.

If you're interested in learning more about hearing and brain health, I've recently developed an online Hearing & Brain Health Academy, which goes into further detail on the science behind untreated hearing loss, cognitive decline and what can be done about it. It's a combination of live seminars and interview content that expands on many of the hearing and brain health concepts introduced in this book.

You'll discover:

- The critical importance of preserving the neural pathways between the ears and the brain

- What science is telling us about dementia prevention

- The mechanics of hearing, how the brain receives and processes sounds, and what causes hearing loss

- How to prevent or overcome social isolation and maintain or restore your quality of life

- Why the term 'use it or lose it' applies to the

connection between hearing and the brain

You can access the academy free of charge by scanning the QR code below or by simply visiting https://neuaudio.link/brainhealth

Supplement

HEARING HEALTH
FOR CAMBODIA

*"True humanity is not thinking less of yourself;
it is thinking of yourself less."*

~CS Lewis

I've been supporting hearing charity All Ears Cambodia since 2012, both as a guest lecturer and hearing device donor. Less than one percent of Cambodians who need hearing aids have them, primarily due to cost. Cambodia remains one of the poorest and most disease-afflicted nations.

All Ears Cambodia is a small, non-governmental audiology charity based in Phnom Penh. What makes them unique is their focus on training local clinicians. Unlike other charities that fly in and out of third-world countries as a once off, the training and employment of local clinicians enables continuity of care, which makes a real difference over the long term.

If you have preloved hearing devices lying around your home, or know someone that has them, please post or drop them into us. We'll fix them up and send them to Cambodia where we're confident they will get used.

Recommended Reading

Atomic Habits, James Clear

Becoming Supernatural: How Common People Are Doing the Uncommon, Dr. Joe Dispenza

Bold, Steven Kottler and Peter Diamandis

End of Alzheimer's, Dr. Dale Bredesen

Flourish, Dr. Martin E.P. Seligman

Flow: The Psychology of Optimal Experience, Dr. Mihaly Csikszentmihályi

Game Changers: What Leaders, Innovators and Mavericks Do to Win at Life, Dave Asprey

Hearing & Brain Health: Startling links between untreated hearing loss and cognitive decline. Andrew Campbell

Homo Deus: A brief history of tomorrow, Yuval Harari

Lifespan, Dr. David Sinclair

Man's Search for Meaning, Dr. Victor Frankl

Mindset: The New Psychology of Success, Carol S. Dweck

The Art of Impossible, Steven Kottler

The Brain that Changes Itself, Norman Doidge

The Science and Technology of Growing Young, Sergey Young

The Science Behind Tapping: A Proven Stress Management Technique for the Mind and Body, Dr. Peta Stapleton

The Village Effect, Susan Pinker

The 1% Rule, Tommy Baker

Tools of Titans: The Tactics, Routines, and Habits of Billionaires, Icons, and World-Class Performers, Tim Ferris

Sapiens: The Pillars of Civilization, Yuval Harari

Academic References

Andersson G, Melin L, Scott B, Lindberg P. An evaluation of a behavioural treatment approach to hearing impairment. Behavior Research Therapy. 1995; 33:283–292

Armstrong NM, An Y, Doshi J, et al. Association of midlife hearing impairment with late-life temporal lobe volume loss. JAMA Otolaryngol Head Neck Surg 2019; 145: 794.

Amieva H, Ouvrard C, Giulioli C, Meillon C, Rullier L, Dartigues JF. Self-reported hearing loss, hearing aids, and cognitive decline in elderly adults: a 25-year study. J Am Geriatric Soc 2015; 63: 2099–104.

Amieva H, Ouvrard C, Meillon C, Rullier L, Dartigues JF. Death, depression, disability, and dementia associated with self-reported hearing problems: a 25-year study. J Gerontol A Biol Sci Med Sci 2018; 73: 1383–89

Barker F, Mackenzie E, Elliott L, Jones S, de Lusignan S. Interventions to improve hearing aid use in adult auditory rehabilitation. Cochrane Database Syst Rev. 2014 Jul 12;(7)

Beck DL. Inside the research: Auditory deprivation, brain changes secondary to hearing loss, and more: An interview with Anu Sharma, PhD. Hearing Review. 2017;24(1):40

Bell L, Wagels L, Neuschaefer-Rube C, Fels J, Gur RE, Konrad K. The Cross-Modal Effects of Sensory Deprivation on Spatial and Temporal Processes in Vision and Audition: A Systematic Review on Behavioral and Neuroimaging

Research since 2000. Neural Plast. 2019; 2019:9603469

Bernabei R, Bonuccelli U, Maggi S, et al, and the participants in the Workshop on Hearing Loss and Cognitive Decline in Older Adults. Hearing loss and cognitive decline in older adults: questions and answers. Aging Clin Exp Res 2014; 26: 567–73

Berman M.G., Jonides J., Kaplan S. The Cognitive Benefits of Interacting with Nature. First Published December 1, 2008 Research Article Find in PubMed https://doi.org/10.1111/j.1467-9280.2008.02225

Blustein, J., and B. E. Weinstein. 2016b. "Blustein and Weinstein Respond" to the Letter by Stein, Z.A., "The Hearing Aid Industry Is More Helpful than Suggested." American Journal of Public Health 106: e1

Brinke L.F., Bolandzadeh N., Nagamatsu L.S., Hsu C.L., Davis, J.C., Miran-Khan K., Liu-Ambrose T., , Department of Physical Therapy, UBC, Vancouver, BC, Canada V6T 1Z3, Aerobic exercise increases hippocampal volume in older women with probable mild cognitive impairment: a 6-month randomised controlled trial. Randomized Controlled Trial. Br J Sports Med. 2015 Feb;49(4):248-54. DOI: 10.1136/bjsports-2013-093184. Epub 2014 Apr 7

Cabral J, Tonocchi R, Ribas Â, Almeida G, Rosa M, Massi G, Berberian AP. The efficacy of hearing aids for emotional and auditory tinnitus issues. Int Tinnitus J. 2016 Jul 22;20(1):54-8

Carniel CZ, Sousa JCF, Silva CDD, Fortunato-Queiroz CAU, Hyppolito MÂ, Santos PLD. Implications of using the hearing aids on quality of life of elderly codas. 2017 Oct 19;29(5)

Caselli G, Lipsi RM. Survival differences among the oldest old in Sardinia: who, what, where, and why. Demographic Research. 2006;14:267–294

Chen Z, Yuan W. Central plasticity and dysfunction elicited by aural deprivation in the critical period. Front Neural Circuits. 2015; 9:26. Published 2015 Jun 2

Cheung SW, Bonham BH, Schreiner CE, Godey B, Copenhaver DA. Realignment of interaural cortical maps in asymmetric hearing loss. J Neurosci 2009; 29: 7065–78

Church, Dawson et al. Epigenetic effects of PTSD remediation in veterans using clinical Emotional Freedom Techniques: A randomized controlled pilot study. American Journal of Health Promotion 32, no. 1 (2018): 112–122. DIO:10.1177/0890117116661154.

Darrow, K. Stop Living in Isolation: How Treating Hearing Loss & Tinnitus can change your life, maintain your independence, and may reduce your risk of dementia. 2017.

Deal JA, Betz J, Yaffe K, et al, for the Health ABC Study Group. Hearing impairment and incident dementia and cognitive decline in older adults: the Health ABC Study. J Gerontol A Biol Sci Med Sci 2016; published online April 12.

Deal JA, Sharrett AR, Albert MS, et al. Hearing impairment and cognitive decline: a pilot study conducted within the atherosclerosis risk in community's neurocognitive study. Am J Epidemiol 2015; 181: 680–90

Fortunato, S., F. Forli, V. Guglielmi, G. Paludetti, S. Berrentini, and A.R. Fetoni. 2016. "A Review of New insights on the association between hearing loss and cognitive decline in ageing." Acta Otorhinolaryngolica Italica 36:155–166

Fritze T, Teipel S, Óvári A, Kilimann I, Witt G, Doblhammer G. Hearing impairment affects dementia incidence. An analysis based on longitudinal health claims data in Germany. PLoS One 2016

Garnefski N, Kraaij V. Cognitive coping and goal adjustment are associated with symptoms of depression and anxiety in people with acquired hearing loss. International Journal of Audiology. 2012; 51:545–550

Garraghty PE, Kaas JH. Neuroplasticity of the adult primate auditory cortex following cochlear hearing loss Am J Otol 1993; 14: 252–58

Gatehouse S. Rehabilitation: identification of needs, priorities and expectations, and the evaluation of benefit. International Journal of Audiology. 2003;42:77–83

Gates GA, Beiser A, Rees TS, D'Agostino RB, Wolf PA. Central auditory dysfunction may precede the onset of clinical dementia in people with probable Alzheimer's disease. J Am Geriatr Soc 2002; 50: 482–88

Gates GA. Central presbycusis: an emerging view. Otolaryngol Head Neck Surg 2012; 147: 1–2

Gates GA, Cobb JL, Linn RT, Rees T, Wolf PA, D'Agostino RB. Central auditory dysfunction, cognitive dysfunction, and dementia in older people. Arch Otolaryngol Head Neck Surg 1996; 122: 161–67

Glick HA, Sharma A. Cortical neuroplasticity and cognitive function in early-stage, mild-moderate hearing loss:

Evidence of neurocognitive benefit from hearing aid use. Front Neurosci. 2020; 14:93

Golub JS, Brickman AM, Ciarleglio AJ, Schupf N, Luchsinger JA. Association of subclinical hearing loss with cognitive performance. JAMA Otolaryngol Head Neck Surg 2019; 146: 57–6.

Gopinath B, Wang JJ, Schneider J, et al. Depressive symptoms in older adults with hearing impairments: the Blue Mountains Study. J Am Geriatr Soc 2009; 57: 1306–08

Gurgel RK, Ward PD, Schwartz S, Norton MC, Foster NL, Tschanz JT. Relationship of hearing loss and dementia: a prospective, population-based study. Otol Neurotol 2014; 35: 775–81

Hallberg LRM, Hallberg U, Kramer SE. Self-reported hearing difficulties, communication strategies and psychological general well-being (quality of life) in patients with acquired hearing impairment. Disability and Rehabilitation. 2008;30:203–212

Hartley D, Rochtchina E, Newall P, Golding M, Mitchell P. Use of hearing aids and assistive listening devices in an older Australian population. J Am Acad Audiol 2010; 21: 642–53

Hölzel, B.K., Carmody J. Vangela M., Congleton C., Yerramsetti S.M., Gard T., &. Lazara S.W.; Mindfulness practice leads to increases in regional brain gray matter density. PMCID: PMC3004979 NIHMSID: NIHMS232587 PMID: 21071182 Psychiatry Res. 2011 Jan 30; 191(1): 36–43. Published online 2010 Nov 10. doi: 10.1016/j.pscychresns.2010.08.006

Hong T, Mitchell P, Burlutsky G, Liew G, Wang JJ. Visual impairment, hearing loss and cognitive function in an older population: Longitudinal findings from the Blue Mountains Eye Study. PLoS One 2016; 11: e0147646

Huang CQ, Dong BR, Lu ZC, Yue JR, Liu QX. Chronic diseases and risk for depression in old age: a meta-analysis of published literature. Ageing Res Rev 2010; 9: 131–41

Kaplan-Neeman R, Muchnik C, Hildesheimer M, Henkin Y. Hearing aid satisfaction and use in the advanced digital era. Laryngoscope. 2012 Sep;122(9):2029-36

Kiely KM, Gopinath B, Mitchell P, Luszcz M, Anstey KJ. Cognitive, health, and sociodemographic predictors of longitudinal decline in hearing acuity among older adults. J Gerontol A Biol Sci Med Sci 2012; 67: 997–1003

Kochkin, S. MarkeTrak VII: Hearing Loss Population Tops 31 Million People, The Hearing Review, Vol. 12(7) July 2005, pp. 16-29. Download: http://www.betterhearing.org/pdfs/MarkeTrak7_Koch kin_July05.pdf

Kochkin, S. & Rogin, C. Quantifying the Obvious: The Impact of Hearing Aids on Quality of Life, The Hearing Review, Vol 7(1) January 2000, pp. 8-34. Download: http://www.betterhearing.org/pdfs/ MR40.pdf

Lin FR, Metter EJ, O'Brien RJ, Resnick SM, Zonderman AB, Ferrucci L. Hearing loss and incident dementia. Arch Neurol 2011; 68: 214–20

Gallacher J, Ilubaera V, Ben-Shlomo Y, et al. Auditory threshold, phonologic demand, and incident dementia. Neurology 2012

Lazar S.W., Catherine E.K, Wasserman, R.H. Jeremy R. Gray, D.N. Greve, D. Treadway M.T., Metta A. McGarvey,E., Quinn B.T., Dusek, J.A. Herbert Benson,F.G., Rauch S.L., Christopher A., Moore, H.l., & Fischld B. Meditation experience is associated with increased cortical thickness. PMCID: PMC1361002 NIHMSID: NIHMS6696 PMID: 16272874

Lenze E.J. MD, Bowie C.R. PhD, Cognitive training for older adults: What works? First published: 18 January 2018 https://doi.org/10.1111/jgs.15230

Lin FR, Ferrucci L, Metter EJ, An Y, Zonderman AB, Resnick SM. Hearing loss and cognition in the Baltimore Longitudinal Study of Aging. Neuropsychology 2011; 25: 763–70

Lin FR. Hearing loss and cognition among older adults in the United States. J Gerontol A Biol Sci Med Sci 2011; 66: 1131–36

Lin MY, Gutierrez PR, Stone KL, et al, and the Study of Osteoporotic Fractures Research Group. Vision impairment and combined vision and hearing impairment predict cognitive and functional decline in older women. J Am Geriatr Soc 2004; 52: 1996–2002

Lin FR, Albert M. Hearing loss and dementia—who is listening? Aging Ment Health 2014; 18: 671–73. Livingston G, Sommerlad A, Orgeta V, et al. Dementia prevention, intervention, and care. Lancet. 2017;390(10113)

Livingston G, Huntley J, Sommerlad A, et al. Dementia prevention, intervention, and care: 2020 report of the Lancet Commission. Lancet. 2020 Aug 8;396

Long P, Wan G, Roberts MT, Corfas G. Myelin development, plasticity, and pathology in the auditory system. Dev

Neurobiol. 2018;78(2)

Loughrey DG, Kelly ME, Kelley GA, Brennan S, Lawlor BA. Association of age-related hearing loss with cognitive function, cognitive impairment, and dementia: a systematic review and meta-analysis. JAMA Otolaryngol Head Neck Surg 2018

Maharaj, M. E. "Differential gene expression after Emotional Freedom Techniques (EFT) treatment: A novel pilot protocol for salivary mRNA assessment." Energy Psychology: Theory, Research, and Treatment 8, no.1 (2016): 17–32. doi:10.9769/EPJ.2016.8.1.MM

Maharani A, Dawes P, Nazroo J, Tampubolon G, Pendleton N. Longitudinal relationship between hearing aid use and cognitive function in older Americans. J Am Geriatr Soc 2018; 66: 1130–36

Mandolesi L., Polverino A., Montuori S., Foti F., Ferraioli G., Sorrentino P., & Sorrentino G. Effects of physical exercise on cognitive functioning and wellbeing: Biological and psychological benefits. Frontiers in Psycholigy, 2018; 9: 509 PMCID: PMC5934999 PMID: 29755380

MacLean C.R., Walton K.G., Wenneberg S.R., Levitsky D.K., Mandarino J.P., Waziri R., Hillis S.L., Schneider R.H., Effects of the Transcendental Meditation program on adaptive mechanisms: changes in hormone levels and responses to stress after 4 months of practice, Clinical Trial: Psychoneuroendocrinology. 1997 May; 22:277-95. DOI: 10.1016/s0306-4530(97)00003-6

McCoy SL, Tun PA, Cox LC, Colangelo M, Stewart RA,

Wingfield A. Hearing loss and perceptual effort: downstream effects on older adults' memory for speech. Q J Exp Psychol A 2005; 58: 22–33

Mondelli MF, Souza PJ. Quality of life in elderly adults before and after hearing aid fitting. Braz J Otorhinolaryngol. 2012 Jun;78(3):49-56

Newby Jill M., Kathleen O'Moore, Samantha Tang, Helen Christensen, Kate Faasse, Acute mental health responses during the COVID-19 pandemic in Australia, July 28, 2020, Plos One journal

Oschman J.L., Chevalier G., & Brown R. The effects of grounding (earthing) on inflammation, the immune response, wound healing, and prevention and treatment of chronic inflammatory and autoimmune diseases PMCID: PMC4378297 PMID: 25848315

Pereira-Jorge M.R, et al. Anatomical and functional MRI changes after one year of auditory rehabilitation with hearing aids. Neural Plasticity. 2018 Sep; 9303674

Pienaar E, Stearn N, Swanepoel de W. Self-reported outcomes of aural rehabilitation for adult hearing aid users in a South African context. S Afr J Commun Disord. 2010 Dec;57:4, 6, 8

Poulain M, Pes G, Salaris L. A population where men live as long as women: Villagrande Strisaili, Sardinia. J Aging Res. 2011;2011:153756

Ray J, Popli G, Fell G. Association of cognition and age-related hearing impairment in the English longitudinal study of ageing. JAMA Otolaryngol Head Neck Surg 2018; 144:

876–82

Rezende BA, Lemos SMA, Medeiros AM. Quality of life of children with poor school performance: association with hearing abilities and behavioral issues Arq Neuropsiquiatr. 2019 Mar;77(3):147-154.

Ribeiro UASL, Souza VC, Lemos SMA Quality of life and social determinants in individual hearing AIDS users codas. 2019 Apr 1;31(2).

Scholes S, Mindell J. Health Survey for England 2014: health, social care and lifestyles. In: Craig R, Fuller E, Mindell J, eds. Chapter 4: Hearing. London: Health and Social Care Information Centre, 2014

Sharma A, Glick H. Cortical neuroplasticity in hearing loss: Why it matters in clinical decision-making for children and adults. Hearing Review. 2018;25(7):20-24

Sinha UK, Hollen KM, Rodriguez R, Miller CA. Auditory system degeneration in Alzheimer's disease. Neurology 1993; 43: 779–85

Subramanian SV, Kim D, Kawachi I. Covariation in the socioeconomic determinants of self rated health and happiness: a multivariate multilevel analysis of individuals and communities in the USA. J Epidemiol Community Health. 2005;59(8):664-669

Bak T.H., Nissan J.J., Allerhand M.M. & Deary I.J. Does bilingualism influence cognitive aging? Annals of Neurology, June 2, 2014 DOI: 10.1002/ana.24158

Valentijn SAM, van Boxtel MPJ, van Hooren SAH, et al.

Change in sensory functioning predicts change in cognitive functioning: results from a 6-year follow-up in the maastricht aging study. J Am Geriatr Soc 2005; 53: 374–80

Verghese J, M.D., Lipton R.B., M.D., Katz M.J , M.P.H., Hall C.B., Ph.D., Derby C.A., Ph.D., Kuslansky G., Ph.D., Ambrose A.F., M.D., Sliwinski M, Ph.D., & Buschke H., M.D. Leisure activities and the risk of dementia in the elderly, June 19, 2003 New England Journal of Medicine, 2003; 348:2508-2516 DOI: 10.1056/NEJMoa022252

Marian V. Ph.D. PMCID & Shook A. The cognitive benefits of being bilingual PMC3583091 PMID: 23447799, 2012 Sep-Oct; 2012: 13. Published online 2012 Oct 31

Waldinger RJ, Schulz MS. What's love got to do with it? Social functioning, perceived health, and daily happiness in married octogenarians. Psychol Aging. 2010;25(2):422-431

Wong Y Joel, Owen Jesse, Gabana Nicole T, Brown, Joshua, McInnis Sydney, Toth Paul, Gilman Lynn. Does gratitude writing improve the mental health of psychotherapy clients? PubMed, 2018 Mar;28 :192-202. DOI: 10.1080/10503307.2016.1169332

WHO. 2017 "Global Costs of Unaddressed Hearing Loss and Cost-Effectiveness of Interventions." A WHO Report, 2017. Geneva: World Health Organization. Licence: CC BY-NC-SA 3.0 IGO.

For more information on blueberries and lion's mane supplements

https://examine.com/supplements/blueberry/
https://examine.com/supplements/lionsmane/

ACKNOWLEDGEMENTS

A big thanks to my talented team and to those who have inspired this book including Samantha Brooks, Joanne Campbell, Michael Collas-Smith, Dr. Keith Darrow, Professor Louise Hickson, Peter Hutson, Anya Hutson, Jeanette Leigh, Brian James, Dr. Doug Maher, Jeffrey Pang and Nicole Turley.

www.ingramcontent.com/pod-product-compliance
Lightning Source LLC
Chambersburg PA
CBHW052011030426
42334CB00029BA/3174